ICU RECALL

RECALL SERIES EDITOR

LORNE H. BLACKBOURNE, M.D.
General Surgeon
Major, Medical Corps
United States Army
Fort Eustis, Virginia

ICU RECALL

Senior Editor

CURTIS G. TRIBBLE, M.D
Professor
Division of Thoracic and Cardiovascular Surgery
University of Virginia Health Sciences Center
Charlottesville, Virginia

Editor

JEFFREY T. COPE, M.D.
Resident in Surgery
University of Virginia School of Medicine
Charlottesville, Virginia

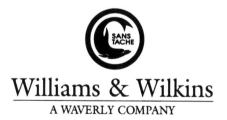

Williams & Wilkins

A WAVERLY COMPANY

BALTIMORE • PHILADELPHIA • LONDON • PARIS • BANGKOK
BUENOS AIRES • HONG KONG • MUNICH • SYDNEY • TOKYO • WROCLAW

Editor: Elizabeth A. Nieginski
Manager, Development Editing: Julie Scardiglia
Managing Editor: Amy G. Dinkel
Marketing Manager: Rebecca Himmelheber
Production Coordinator: Felecia R. Weber
Illustration Planner: Felecia R. Weber
Cover Designer: Karen Klinedinst
Typesetter: Port City Press, Inc.
Printer: Port City Press, Inc.
Digitized Illustrations: Port City Press, Inc.
Binder: Port City Press, Inc.

Copyright ©1997 Williams & Wilkins

351 West Camden Street
Baltimore, Maryland 21201-2436 USA

Rose Tree Corporate Center
1400 North Providence Road
Building II, Suite 5025
Media, Pennsylvania 19063-2043 USA

Accurate indications, adverse reactions and dosage schedules for drugs are provided in this book, but it is possible that they may change. The reader is urged to review the package information data of the manufacturers of the medications mentioned.

Printed in the United States of America

First Edition

Library of Congress Cataloging-in-Publication Data
Tribble, Curtis G.
ICU recall / Curtis G. Tribble
    p.   cm.
Includes index.
ISBN 0-683-08408-9
1. Critical care medicine—Examinations, questions, etc. I. Title.
[DNLM: 1. Intensive Care Units—examination questions. 2. Critical care—examination questions. WX 18.2 T822i 1997]
RC86.9.T75 1997
616'.028'076—dc21
DNLM/DLC
for Library of Congress   96-49031
                                                                      CIP

The publishers have made every effort to trace the copyright holders for borrowed material. If they have inadvertently overlooked any, they will be pleased to make the necessary arrangements at the first opportunity.

To purchase additional copies of this book, call our customer service department at **(800) 638-0672** or fax orders to **(800) 447-8438.** For other book services, including chapter reprints and large quantity sales, ask for the Special Sales department.

Canadian customers should call **(800) 665-1148,** or fax **(800) 665-0103.** For all other calls originating outside of the United States, please call **(410) 528-4223** or fax us at **(410) 528-8550.**

Visit *Williams & Wilkins* on the Internet: http://www.wwilkins.com or contact our customer service department at **custserv@wwilkins.com.** Williams & Wilkins customer service representatives are available from 8:30 am to 6:00 pm, EST, Monday through Friday, for telephone access.

98 99 00
2 3 4 5 6 7 8 9 10

CONTRIBUTING AUTHORS

Reid B. Adams, M.D.
Assistant Professor of Surgery
University of Virginia School of Medicine
Charlottesville, Virginia

James D. Bergin, M.D.
Associate Professor of Medicine
University of Virginia School of Medicine
Charlottesville, Virginia

Eugene F. Foley, M.D.
Assistant Professor of Surgery
University of Virginia School of Medicine
Charlottesville, Virginia

Robert Hannan, M.D.
Associate Professor of Surgery
University of Virginia School of Medicine
Charlottesville, Virginia

Michael Ishitani, M.D.
Assistant Professor of Surgery
University of Virginia School of Medicine
Charlottesville, Virginia

William Killinger, M.D.
Thoracic Surgeon
Raleigh, North Carolina

Ryan Lesh, M.D.
Assistant Professor of Anesthesiology
University of Virginia School of Medicine
Charlottesville, Virginia

George Leisure, M.D.
Assistant Professor of Anesthesiology
University of Virginia School of Medicine
Charlottesville, Virginia

Alan Matsumoto, M.D.
Associate Professor of Radiology
University of Virginia School of Medicine
Charlottesville, Virginia

Eugene D. McGahren, M.D.
Assistant Professor of Surgery
University of Virginia School of Medicine
Charlottesville, Virginia

Katherine Michael, Pharm.D.
Pharmacy Clinical Specialist
University of Virginia School of Medicine
Charlottesville, Virginia

John S. Minasi, M.D.
Assistant Professor of Surgery
University of Virginia School of Medicine
Charlottesville, Virginia

George Rich, M.D.
Assistant Professor of Anesthesiology
University of Virginia School of Medicine
Charlottesville, Virginia

Karen Schwenzer, M.D.
Associate Professor of Surgery
University of Virginia School of Medicine
Charlottesville, Virginia

Craig Slingluff, M.D.
Associate Professor of Surgery
University of Virginia School of Medicine
Charlottesville, Virginia

Burkhard Spiekermann, M.D.
Assistant Professor of Anesthesiology
University of Virginia School of Medicine
Charlottesville, Virginia

J. Benjamin Tribble, M.D.
General Surgeon
Columbia, South Carolina

David E. Tribble, M.D.
Thoracic Surgeon
Columbia, South Carolina

Reid W. Tribble, M.D.
Thoracic Surgeon
Columbia, South Carolina

Jeffrey S. Young, M.D.
Assistant Professor of Surgery
University of Virginia School of Medicine
Charlottesville, Virginia

CONTRIBUTORS

The following contributed to this book while they were medical students at the University of Virginia School of Medicine.

John Connors, M.D.
Matt Edwards, M.D.
Ryan Herrington, M.D.
Steve Kim, M.D.

Scott Ross, M.D.
John Sperling, M.D.
Blake VanMeter, M.D.
Kent Weathers, M.D.

The following contributed to this book while they were surgery residents at the University of Virginia School of Medicine.

Scott Arnold, M.D.
Christopher Bartels, M.D.
Oliver Binns, M.D.
Lorne H. Blackbourne, M.D.
Osbert Blow, M.D.
Scott A. Buchanan, M.D.
Barry Chan, M.D.
Gerald Cephus, M.D.
Richard Earnhart, M.D.
David Graham, M.D.

Nancy Harthun, M.D.
John Kern, M.D.
Christopher King, M.D.
Lisa King, M.D.
Michael C. Mauney, M.D.
Addison May, M.D.
Lynn Rosenlof, M.D.
Robert Sawyer, M.D.
Donald Schmit, M.D.
Michael Towler, M.D.

The following contributed to this book while they were surgery residents at Roanoke Memorial Hospital, Roanoke, Virginia.

Steve Thies, M.D.
Tim Edmiston, M.D.
Joseph Bianchi, M.D.

Contents

SECTION 3
PATHOLOGIC PROCESSES IN THE ICU

SECTION 4
PATIENT-SPECIFIC CONSIDERATIONS IN THE ICU

Preface

ICU Recall is an outgrowth of the earlier effort at the University of Virginia in writing *Surgical Recall* and *Advanced Surgical Recall.* Medical students, residents, and faculty members at the University of Virginia, allied with the Department of Surgery, have written most of the questions in this guide. Our goal is to provide young trainees with concise information about intensive care unit issues.

Section 1

Overview and Background ICU Information

1   Introduction

USING THE STUDY GUIDE

This study guide is based on the premise that knowing the right questions is at least as important as knowing the answers. In fact, a case could be made that knowing the right questions is *more* important than knowing the answers. All medical students are taught that at least half of what they learn in medical school will be outdated within 5 years, and this process will only accelerate with time. However, it is the answers that change, not the questions.

The primary reason for the format used in this study guide is that people learn better when questioned than when lectured to. In a sense, this approach goes back to the tradition of Socrates, and it has been perpetuated in medicine as much as anywhere else in Western education.

The guide is used most effectively when you cover the answers while posing the questions to yourself. This book is designed so that it can be carried around in your pocket, allowing you to take advantage of the scraps of time that inevitably accrue during a clinical day. Because each of the questions is relatively self-contained, very small bits of time can be used efficiently in this way. Some readers have even found it useful to tear these books up into portions to make them all the more portable.

ICU NOTES

There are two approaches to note writing in the ICU. One is what some have called the "timed approach." Using this approach, a person will sit down and rather instinctively write a note in the chart until a certain amount of time (determined subconsciously) has elapsed. Usually, that person will make a pretense in the ICU of writing an organ-system type of note.

The other approach, which contrasts with the timed system, is the "checklist approach." This is analogous to the use of a checklist by a pilot taking off in a commercial jetliner. Pilots are required to have a checklist that they review to make sure that they have addressed each issue before takeoff. There is no reason not to use this approach in the ICU because, when you are writing these notes, you may be somewhat tired and possibly distracted by all the urgent issues that can arise even while you are writing notes. A sample checklist follows. However, you should add to and subtract from this list as you see fit.
neuro
    mental status, pain, pain relief
    neuro checks, neuro deficits
    psych, consults, meds
    ETOH, DT precautions

seizures, seizure meds
respiratory
  respiratory distress, ABGs, vent settings
  exam, CXR
  bronchodilators, meds, levels
CVS
  BP, P, rhythm, ectopy, EKGs
  CV meds, drips, levels, digoxin
  cardiac enzymes
renal
  fluid status, UOP, wt, IVFs (type and rate)
  I&O, CVP, CXR fluid, BUN, Cr, Foley
  lytes, Ca^{++}, Mg^{++}, $PO_4 \equiv$
  acid–base status
  dialysis
GI
  bowel fxn, gas, nausea, diet
  NGT, H_2 blockers, OBR, lactulose
  liver fxn, LFTs, PT, bilirubin
  panc fxn, amylase, panc enzymes
endo
  DM: glc, DU's, insulin
  thyroid, TFTs, synthroid
  adrenals, steroids, adrenal insufficiency
heme
  hct, transfusions, blood in bank
  clotting studies, vitK, SQ heparin
ID
  temp, Tmax, WBC
  cultures, sensitivities, abx, abx levels
  CXR, UA, lines
nutrition
  TPN, tube feedings, PO intake
  lipids, trace elements, vitamins
  N_2 balance, wt increase, visceral proteins
wounds
  appearance of wounds, debridement
  drains, dsg changes
  review traumatic injuries of multiple trauma victims
meds
  list
path
  reports of all tissues sent to path
impression
  list all issues, problems, and impressions
plan
  have a plan that addresses each of the issues listed in your impression

2 _____

Overall ICU Environment

What should be your overall relationship to the rest of the health care team?

All who work together in the care of ICU patients are teammates. There are no unimportant teammates. Those who provide ancillary care make it possible for you to be a physician. Many of these people, including respiratory therapists, nurses, and perfusionists, will function practically as colleagues.

What should be the role of the medical student in the care of an ICU patient?

Medical students should view themselves as their patients' "main" doctors. In essence, using the more senior members of the team as consultants, students should take particular responsibility for information gathering and note writing, as well as communicating with families, reviewing studies, and participating in procedures.

What types of things can be considered unimportant in the ICU?

There are no unimportant details. *Everything* matters. Nothing is neutral. Virtually everything that goes on in the ICU will either help or hinder your patient. Even things as subtle as the noise level, the temperature, the light, music, as well as the more obvious details of laboratory values, medicines, and procedures can be critical to a patient's outcome.

How does one determine a patient's level of awareness in the ICU?

You should assume that patients will hear, see, and feel everything that is said about them and done to them. This ethic should be carried from rounds, to procedures, to discussions with the family. This concept should even be extrapolated to the point where both the health care team and the family should be encouraged to talk to the patients, recognizing that you can never be certain how much the patient will know at any given time. Sooner or later, you will be astonished by how much patients remember from their ICU experiences.

3   Ethical Issues in the ICU

ETHICAL DECISION MAKING IN THE ICU

How do you decide when to continue or discontinue what may seem like aggressive or even futile therapy?

These decisions should be made jointly by the entire health care team, the patient, and the patient's family.

What is the single most important question you should ask when ethical concerns arise?

Ask yourself whether the benefit of the therapy is worth the burden of the therapy.

Who should have the greatest say in what treatments are instituted or discontinued?

The patient. However, often in the ICU, the patient's immediate wishes cannot be discerned. In this case, the health care team and the family are obligated to make some attempt at determining what the patient's wishes would be. Sometimes there are written guidelines—often, there are not. In the latter instance, your obligation is to try to establish what the patient would want. Thus, the team should not necessarily do what the family or the health care team wants, but rather, what the patient would have wanted.

Are there any other guidelines for helping the health care team discern what sort of recommendations to make to the family under these conditions?

A very useful tenet is to think for yourself what you would want for an analogous member of your own family, whether it be a grandparent, parent, spouse, sibling, or child. Often, this approach is very helpful in considering recommendations and, of course, it has credibility with the patient's family.

EUTHANASIA

What is the definition of euthanasia?	The act of facilitating death without pain for a person suffering from an incurable and painful disease or condition. Translated from the Greek, it means "easy death."
What is the definition of passive euthanasia?	Withdrawing or withholding medical treatment to facilitate painless death
What is the definition of active euthanasia?	Directly intervening to cause death, in a painless fashion, for those who are hopelessly ill *and* in pain
What percentage of ICU physicians have participated in passive euthanasia?	Virtually all physicians who practice in this arena have participated in passive euthanasia.
What European country has a legalized active euthanasia program?	The Netherlands
How many patients are estimated to be actively euthanized each year in this country?	Between 5,000–10,000 patients annually
Which states have had referendums that indicated public approval for legalization of active euthanasia?	The states of Washington and California
Is active euthanasia currently legal in any state in the USA?	No

BRAIN DEATH AND ORGAN TRANSPLANTATION

Before 1968, what were the traditionally accepted criteria for documenting patient death?	Cessation of cardiac and respiratory activity

Who was responsible for establishing these criteria?	William Harvey, in 1627
What were the new criteria for determining death as proposed by the Ad-Hoc Committee of the Harvard Medical School in 1968?	Total and irreversible loss of brain function, or brain death
What new medical technology led to the legislation of brain death criteria?	The increasing use of the mechanical ventilator
What criteria must be met before brain death can be determined?	These are the criteria (which vary slightly from state to state) established by the Uniform Determination of Death Act: 1. Absence of neurologic function 2. Irreversibility of neurologic deficit 3. Apnea 4. Confirmatory tests
What is absence of neurologic function?	Total absence of brain function as indicated by: 1. Unresponsive coma 2. No spontaneous movements of any kind 3. Absence of all brain-stem function
How is irreversibility established?	1. Cause of neurologic deficit should be deemed sufficient to cause irreversible brain death. 2. Exclude hypothermia and/or CNS-acting drugs. 3. No improvement in neurologic exam for 24 hours
What are the standard signs for absence of brain-stem function?	1. Fixed pupils that are unreactive to light 2. Absent corneal, vestibular–ocular, and gag reflexes 3. No motor movements to stimulation of somatic areas within the cranial nerve distribution 4. Absent respiratory movements, with $PaCO_2 > 60$ mm Hg or 20 mm Hg > baseline

What tests confirm the absence of brain-stem reflexes?

1. Corneal: no blink with corneal touch
2. Vestibular: cold caloric stimulation (*doll's eyes*)
3. Oropharyngeal: no gag reflex

What percentage of brain-dead patients will have small pupils?

24%

What percentage of brain-dead patients will have deep tendon or plantar reflexes?

33%

What diagnostic tests can be performed to determine brain death?

1. EEG
2. Cerebral blood flow tests

Are these tests necessary to prove brain death?

No, but they can be used as confirmation in equivocal cases.

Who is absolutely qualified to determine brain death in a patient?

The attending neurologist or neurosurgeon. However, some states do allow other doctors to determine brain death.

What is perhaps the largest impediment to organ transplantation becoming a routine and dependable cure for end-stage organ disease today?

A shortage of donor organs

Is family or surrogate approval mandatory before organ retrieval in a brain-dead patient?

Yes

Is it currently acceptable to retrieve organs for transplantation from a patient who has suffered cardiopulmonary death but has not been declared clinically brain dead?

Yes, if the cessation of cardiac activity is permanent, the family has given permission, and the organs in question are salvageable.

KEY PRINCIPLES OF BIOMEDICAL ETHICS

What is the consequentialist theory of biomedical ethics?	Actions are deemed right or wrong based on their consequences rather than on any inherent characteristic.
What is the deontological theory of biomedical ethics?	Actions are inherently right or wrong before their enactment.
What are the four key biomedical ethical principles that should direct physicians in ethical decision making?	1. Beneficence 2. Nonmaleficence 3. Autonomy 4. Justice
What is the definition of beneficence?	To restore health and relieve pain and suffering ("to do good")
What is the definition of nonmaleficence?	To do no harm (*primum non nocere*)
What is the definition of autonomy?	The right of self-determination (involves respecting the individuality of others)
What is the definition of justice?	The fair allocation of medical resources to all citizens

WITHHOLDING/WITHDRAWING LIFE SUPPORT

What is considered basic life support?	Food, water, and supplemental oxygen
What is considered advanced life support?	Mechanical ventilation, dialysis, inotropic support, pressors, mechanical circulatory support, and critical care
Is it ever appropriate to withhold basic life support?	Yes, when a patient is terminally ill, suffering, and awaiting death. Prolonging basic life support would only prolong patient indignity and suffering.
What percentage of patients undergoing CPR in the hospital survive to leave the hospital?	Approximately 5%

What percentage of patients who undergo CPR in the hospital survive the event?

Approximately 22%

What three criteria help determine medical futility?

1. Disease must be terminal.
2. Disease must be irreversible.
3. Death must be imminent.

Are there guidelines for withdrawing advanced life support?

Yes. When the burden to the patient outweighs the benefit (or the potential benefit)

Who can determine if a patient is legally competent?

In simple cases, most ICU physicians can make this determination. When in doubt, psychiatric consultation is necessary.

Can a legal surrogate be appointed by the court if a patient has no family or legal guardian?

Yes, a team of nurses, physicians, administrators, and religious representatives can be established.

Can a physician or group of physicians legally withdraw life support if the team has determined that continued medical treatment will be futile, but the family or legal surrogate will not consent to this action?

No

LEGAL PRECEDENTS AND LEGISLATION

What case decided by the New Jersey Supreme Court in 1976 determined that "substituted judgments" by a family or legal surrogate were valid in consenting for withdrawal of mechanical ventilation?

The Karen Ann Quinlan case

Which case in 1981 found two California physicians innocent of committing murder when they decided to withdraw basic life support from a terminally ill patient with the consent of the patient's family?

Barber v Superior Court

Which court decision mandated the ability of the patient or legal surrogate to refuse medical therapy necessary to sustain life against the wishes of the physician?

Bartling v Superior Court

What other important ruling was determined by the *Bartling v Superior Court* decision?

Mr. Bartling was deemed legally competent while on the ventilator.

What was the first case to reach the U.S. Supreme Court concerning withdrawing or withholding life support from a legally incompetent patient?

Cruzan v Harmon

What was the ruling?

The U.S. Supreme Court supported the state of Missouri Supreme Court's ruling, which prohibited families from withdrawing life support from an incompetent patient unless there was "clear and convincing" evidence that this was the patient's wish before he or she was incapacitated (living will).

What document allows a family or legal guardian to determine the type of health care a patient can receive if he or she is deemed incompetent?

An advanced directive, or living will

What three types of living will legislation exist?	1. Generic living will 2. Natural death act directives 3. Durable Power of Attorney for Health Care
Which type of living will is most consistently recognized as valid by state legislations?	The Durable Power of Attorney for Health Care
What does this will do?	It appoints an "attorney in fact," who is empowered to make medical decisions for the patient if he or she becomes legally incompetent.
What Act passed in 1990 by the U.S. Congress supported the use of advance directives?	The Patient Self-Determination Act
What did this Act require of health care providers?	1. Provide information to patients about advance directives at the time of admission. 2. Document whether advanced directives had been executed. 3. Educate the health care staff and community about advance directives.
What are advance directives?	Documents stating the desires of the patient regarding specific treatments that should be either withheld or rendered in the event that the patient becomes seriously ill in the future

CONSENT

What is informed consent?	The patient has been counseled on his/her condition, options for treatment, risks and benefits of each option, and has chosen for himself or herself an appropriate course of action.
If the patient is unable to provide consent and no next of kin is available, what is needed to perform an emergency procedure?	A note must be written in the hospital chart, stating the emergent need for a lifesaving procedure and bearing the signature of two treating physicians.

Who can provide consent for an adult patient who is unable to consent for himself or herself?

Priority for consent by next of kin:
1. The spouse
2. An adult son or daughter
3. One parent
4. An adult brother or sister
5. A legally appointed guardian of the patient at the time of consent

4

ICU Pharmacology

THROMBOLYTIC AGENTS

How do they work?	Directly or indirectly convert plasminogen to plasmin, thus inducing clot lysis
Available agents?	1. Streptokinase (SK) 2. Urokinase (UK) 3. Alteplase (rTPA) 4. Anistreplase (APSAC)
Indications?	1. Early (within 6–12 hrs) treatment of acute MI 2. Treatment of acute deep vein thrombosis (DVT) and pulmonary edema (PE) in selected patients 3. Intra-arterial infusion for occluded arteries or vascular grafts 4. Clearance of occluded infusion catheters (UK only)
Absolute contraindications (major risk for bleeding or allergic reaction)?	1. Active bleeding 2. Recent (within 6 weeks) trauma, surgery, head injury, or intracranial event 3. CPR > 10 minutes with evidence of chest wall injury 4. Treatment with SK or APSAC in the preceding 6 months, or recent streptococcal infection (in these cases may still use rTPA or UK) 5. Pregnancy 6. Uncontrolled hypertension 7. Intracranial neoplasm 8. Aortic dissection 9. Pericarditis
Adverse reactions?	1. Bleeding 2. Hypotension 3. Anaphylaxis (SK and APSAC) 4. Reperfusion arrhythmias

ANTIARRHYTHMIC AND RATE-CONTROLLING AGENTS

LIDOCAINE

Indications?	Ventricular tachycardia; prevention of recurrent ventricular fibrillation after resuscitation
Dosing?	1. Loading dose: 1–1.5 mg/kg total body weight (usually 100 mg). Repeat 1/2 loading dose at 15 minutes to account for rapid distribution. 2. Infusion: 1–4 mg/min. Do not need to wean infusion.
Therapeutic serum concentration?	2–5 mg/L
Pharmacokinetics?	1. Plasma half-life—90 minutes 2. Metabolism: 90% hepatic, liver blood-flow dependent clearance (decreased clearance with CHF, MI, cimetidine, propranolol, advanced age). Active metabolites may accumulate with renal dysfunction. 3. Protein binding: 70% bound to α-1-acid glycoprotein (May need higher concentration the first 24 hours post-MI due to increased binding.)
Adverse effects?	Dose-related CNS effects (paresthesias, psychosis, lethargy, seizures); dose-related cardiac depression (bradycardia, sinus arrest, hypotension, myocardial depression)

PROCAINAMIDE (PA)

Indications?	1. Treatment of ventricular and supraventricular tachyarrhythmias 2. Prevents recurrences of atrial fibrillation/flutter
IV dosing?	1. Loading dose: up to 17 mg/kg at a rate of 20–30 mg/min (usually about 1 g to load) 2. Infusion of 2–4 mg/min; do not need to wean infusion.

Therapeutic serum concentration?	PA only: 4–12 mg/L. Total PA + N-acetyl procainamide (NAPA): < 30 mg/L.
Pharmacokinetics?	1. Plasma half-life: 3–5 hours 2. Metabolism: hepatically metabolized to active metabolite (NAPA)
Adverse effects?	1. Cardiac effects: (conduction disturbances, AV block, QT prolongation that may lead to torsades de pointes, hypotension, myocardial depression) 2. GI effects: nausea, vomiting, diarrhea 3. Lupus-like syndrome (with chronic use)

BRETYLIUM

Indications?	1. Drug-resistant ventricular arrhythmias 2. Ventricular fibrillation in cardiac arrest
Dosing?	Loading dose: 5–10 mg/kg (usually 500 mg) over 10–20 minutes. Load may be given rapidly in pulseless patients. Infusion: 2–4 mg/min.
Pharmacokinetics?	Plasma half-life: 7–8 hrs. Excretion: excreted unchanged by the kidneys.
Adverse effects?	1. Hypotension (with rapid infusion) 2. Transient hypertension from norepinephrine release 3. CNS effects 4. Bradycardia 5. Nausea/vomiting with rapid infusion in conscious patients. (*Note:* Should never be used in postop cardiac surgical patients since it can cause profound cardiovascular collapse.)

DIGOXIN

Indications?	Rate control in atrial fibrillation not related purely to catecholamine excess (onset of action several hours).

Dose?

1. Loading dose: 15–20 µg/kg lean body weight (reduce by 25% for uremic patients). Usually load with total of 1 mg. Divide loading dose into 3–4 doses administered at least 2 hours apart (every 4–6 hours preferably) to allow for drug distribution to myocardium and assessment of therapeutic/adverse effects.
2. Maintenance dose: 0.125–0.25 mg/day (adjust for renal dysfunction)

Therapeutic serum concentration?

0.8–2.0 ng/ml (serum level not well correlated with rate control effect)

Pharmacokinetics?

1. Plasma half-life: 36 hours (with normal renal function)
2. Excretion: primarily by the kidney. It is not cleared by dialysis, so be very cautious in uremic patients.
3. Volume of distribution: very large (serum concentration much lower than tissue concentration after distribution). Measure serum concentration at least 6 hours after last dose to avoid false elevation.

Adverse effects?

1. Arrhythmias, conduction disturbances
2. Anorexia, nausea/vomiting/diarrhea
3. Visual disturbances
4. Fatigue, weakness. Maintain serum potassium > 3.5 mEq/ml to lessen risk of toxicity.

Drug interactions?

Procainamide, quinidine, verapamil, amiodarone (all increase digoxin serum concentration)

How may digoxin toxicity be treated in dialysis patients?

The antibody (digibind) to digoxin is given and plasmapheresis may be used to clear the antibody-bound digoxin.

DILTIAZEM

Indications?

Rate control in atrial fibrillation/flutter and paroxysmal supraventricular tachycardia

Dose?

1. Loading dose: 0.25 mg/kg (20 mg) IV push over 2 minutes; may repeat at 0.35 mg/kg (25 mg) in 15 minutes if inadequate response; loading doses of < 0.25 mg/kg less effective
2. Maintenance infusion: 5–15 mg/hr

Conversion to oral therapy?

5 mg/hr = 180 mg/day; 7 mg/hr = 240 mg/day; 11 mg/hr = 360 mg/day

Pharmacokinetics?

1. Plasma half-life: 3–4 hrs; rapid decline in serum concentration after IV bolus; terminal half-life: 3–4 hours
2. Metabolism: hepatically metabolized to inactive metabolites; nonlinear elimination with infusion rates > 15 mg/hr (see discussion of "nonlinear elimination" in pharmacokinetics section)

Adverse reactions?

1. Hypotension, bradycardia
2. Flushing
3. Injection site reactions
4. Caution in combination with IV β-blockers, digoxin, or severe CHF
5. Contraindicated in Wolff-Parkinson-White syndrome (WPW)

VERAPAMIL

Indications?

Rate control in atrial fibrillation/flutter and paroxysmal supraventricular tachycardia (PSVT)

Dose?

Loading dose: 0.075–0.15 mg/kg (2.5–10 mg) IV push over 2 minutes; repeat in 10 minutes if no response; maintenance infusion: 0.005 mg/kg/min

Pharmacokinetics?

1. Onset of action: 2–3 minutes (IV)
2. Plasma half-life: 110 minutes (IV)
3. Hepatically metabolized to active metabolite (norverapamil), which may accumulate in renal dysfunction

Adverse effects?	Hypotension, bradycardia, heart block, CHF; caution with IV β-blockers, digoxin, and severe heart failure; contraindicated in WPW

ADENOSINE

Indications?	1. Rate control and/or conversion of PSVT (including WPW) 2. Initial treatment/diagnosis of wide-complex tachycardia of uncertain type
Dose?	1. 6-mg rapid IV push followed immediately by a 10-ml saline flush (administer centrally and as close to the heart as possible due to rapid degradation) 2. May repeat twice at 12 mg every 2 minutes.
Pharmacokinetics?	1. Plasma half-life: 5–10 seconds (clearance not influenced by renal or hepatic disease) 2. Metabolism: metabolized to inosine and adenosine monophosphate by erythrocytes and vascular endothelial cells
Adverse effects?	1. Transient facial flushing 2. Chest discomfort 3. Dyspnea 4. May cause transient bradycardia or AV block (you will probably see one monitor screen of asystole) 5. Contraindicated in second- or third-degree heart block
Drug interactions?	1. Higher degree AV block with carbamazepine and calcium channel blockers 2. Potentiated by dipyridamole (Persantine) 3. Antagonized by methylxanthines (theophylline, caffeine)

DRUGS USED IN ADVANCED CARDIAC LIFE SUPPORT (ACLS)

EPINEPHRINE

Mechanism of action?

The beneficial effect of epinephrine in cardiac arrest is related to its vasoconstrictive properties and to its inotropic effect, which improves myocardial and cerebral blood flow.

Indications?

Any pulseless rhythm (ventricular fibrillation, asystole, EMD)

Dosage?

1. 1-mg IV push if patient has no measurable blood pressure, every 3–5 minutes may give up to 3–5 mg in patients who fail to respond to lower doses
2. If patient is generating some pressure, do not push all of the 1-mg ampule at once.

Route?

1. Central administration preferred
2. May be given via the endotracheal tube in doses 2–2.5 times the IV dose (dilute in at least 10 ml)
3. If given peripherally, follow with 10–20-ml flush and elevate extremity
4. Can be given as an intracardiac injection if all else fails

Adverse effects?

Arrhythmias, palpitations, angina, hypertension, tissue necrosis if extravasated

ATROPINE

Mechanism of action?

Inhibition of muscarinic action of acetylcholine, resulting in increased heart rate and faster AV nodal conduction

Indications?

1. Symptomatic bradycardia
2. Ventricular asystole

Dose?	0.5–1-mg IV push every 3–5 minutes, up to a maximum of 2 mg
Route?	1. Central administration preferred 2. May be given via the endotracheal tube in doses 2–2.5 times the IV dose (dilute in at least 10 ml of IV fluid) 3. If given peripherally, follow with 10–20-ml flush and elevate extremity
Adverse effects?	1. Paradoxical bradycardia with doses less than 0.5 mg 2. Anticholinergic effects (dry mouth, mydriasis, urinary retention, tachycardia) 3. May precipitate ventricular arrhythmias in patients with myocardial ischemia

MAGNESIUM SULFATE

Mechanism of action?	A primarily intracellular cation, whose deficiency has been shown to precipitate and/or aggravate ventricular arrhythmias. Administration may be beneficial regardless of the pretreatment serum magnesium concentration.
Indications?	1. Treatment of torsades de pointes ventricular tachycardia 2. Treatment of V fib/V tach unresponsive to lidocaine and bretylium 3. Any cardiac arrest situation in which hypomagnesemia is known or suspected. (It is useful to keep the mg on the high side of normal in all cardiac patients. Shown to lessen arrhythmias and improve survival after myocardial infarction.)
Dosage and administration?	For V fib/V tach, 1–2-g IV push over 1–2 minutes; otherwise, 1 g over 15 minutes
Adverse effects if given too quickly?	Hypotension, heart block, asystole, respiratory muscle weakness, hyporeflexia, hypocalcemia

PHARMACOKINETICS AND PHARMACODYNAMICS

What is the difference between pharmacokinetics and pharmacodynamics?

1. Pharmacokinetics—the distribution, metabolism, or elimination (ADME) of a drug
2. Pharmacodynamics—the concentration-related effect of the drug on an organism

What major factors affect the pharmacokinetics of drugs?

1. Renal and hepatic function affect elimination and metabolism.
2. Protein binding and fluid status affect distribution.

What two plasma proteins are most important for protein binding of drugs?

1. Albumin: commonly binds acidic drugs (e.g., phenytoin)
2. α-1-acid glycoprotein: commonly binds basic drugs (e.g., lidocaine)

What parameter is most commonly used to estimate renal function?

Serum creatinine

What factor other than renal function affects serum creatinine in ICU patients?

Patients with decreased muscle mass will have falsely low serum creatinine levels.

How is creatinine clearance determined?

By measuring urine clearance over a 6–24-hour period

What commonly used agents in the ICU require adjustment for renal dysfunction?

1. Antibiotics (especially aminoglycosides)
2. Histamine (H_2) blockers
3. Some sedatives with active metabolites (midazolam, meperidine)

Which laboratory parameters are useful to estimate hepatic function?

There are no reliable indicators of metabolic capacity. In general, bilirubin indicates the liver's ability to conjugate and prothrombin time (PT) indicates the liver's synthetic capacity.

What are the two major types of reactions?

1. Phase I reactions (oxidation, reduction, hydrolysis) usually convert the substances to active metabolites.
2. Phase II reactions (conjugation to form glucuronides, sulfate, or

acetates) usually convert substances to inactive metabolites.

What are common hepatic enzyme inducers?

Carbamazepine, ethanol (chronic), phenobarbital, phenytoin, rifampin, tobacco abuse

What are common hepatic enzyme inhibitors?

Cimetidine, ethanol (acute), erythromycin, ketoconazole, omeprazole, ciprofloxacin, valproic acid

The clearance of which medications commonly used in the ICU are hepatic blood flow-dependent?

Lidocaine, theophylline, and cimetidine

What pharmacokinetic effect explains the large discrepancy between the parenteral and oral doses of drugs (such as propranolol and verapamil)?

First-pass effect, in which an orally administered drug is absorbed into the portal circulation and partially metabolized by the liver before reaching the systemic circulation. First-pass metabolism can account for an up to 100-fold difference in oral and parenteral dose.

What is a half-life?

The time required for the serum concentration of a drug to decrease by one half. This may not always correspond to duration of therapeutic effect.

What is nonlinear elimination?

Enzymes responsible for metabolism become saturated at a certain serum concentration. Above this concentration, increases in doses will result in disproportionate (nonlinear) increases in serum concentrations. The most common example is phenytoin.

What factors in ICU patients most likely explain poor oral and/or IM drug absorption?

Poor tissue perfusion of the GI tract and extremities; ileus

MUSCLE RELAXANTS

What are the sedative or analgesic properties of neuromuscular blockers (NMB)?

None. Patients can be paralyzed and still fully aware of their surroundings.

What are the two classes of NMB?

1. Depolarizing
2. Nondepolarizing

What are the class, onset, and duration of succinylcholine (Sch)?

1. Depolarizing
2. Onset < 1 minute
3. Duration of action 5–10 minutes ($T\frac{1}{2}$ = 3–5 minutes)

What is the primary indication for Sch?

Rapid muscle relaxation for endotracheal intubation

What are the potential side effects of Sch?

1. Hypertension
2. Cardiac arrhythmias
3. Tachycardia or bradycardia
4. Increased intracranial pressure
5. Hyperkalemia (usually a rise of 0.5–1 mEq/L)
6. Prolonged paralysis (in patients with atypical cholinesterase)
7. Malignant hyperthermia
8. Increased intraocular pressure (especially in patients with glaucoma)

Which conditions predispose patients for the greatest risk of Sch-induced hyperkalemia?

1. Burns
2. Massive soft tissue trauma
3. Spinal cord injury
4. Neurologic/neuromuscular disorders
5. Intraperitoneal sepsis
6. Renal failure (possibly)

Is there a window of safety for the use of Sch in patients with acute spinal cord injury?

Yes, in the first 24 hours

What is malignant hyperthermia (MH)?

A genetic (autosomal dominant with variable penetrance) skeletal muscle abnormality that results in a hypermetabolic state when triggered

Which agents trigger MH?	Sch, volatile anesthetics (e.g., halothane, isoflurane, etc.)
What are the manifestations of MH?	1. Trismus/masseter muscle spasm (considered to be premonitory of MH) 2. Hypercapnea (often the first sign to appear) 3. Tachycardia 4. Tachypnea 5. Temperature elevation (1–2° C every 5 minutes) 6. Hypertension 7. Cardiac dysrhythmias 8. Acidosis 9. Hypoxemia 10. Hyperkalemia 11. Skeletal muscle rigidity 12. Myoglobinuria (creatine phosphokinase [CPK] > 20,000 within 12–24 hours) 13. Disseminated intravascular coagulation (DIC)
What is the primary drug for treating MH?	Dantrolene sodium
Name examples of long-acting, intermediate-acting, and relatively short-acting nondepolarizing muscle relaxants (NDMR).	Long-acting: d-tubocurarine (Curare) Intermediate-acting: atracurium, vecuronium, rocuronium Short-acting: mivacurium
Which NDMRs cause a histamine release?	Curare, metocurine, atracurium
What is the effect of this histamine release?	Decreased blood pressure and reflex tachycardia
Which NDMR causes sympathetic nervous system stimulation?	Pancuronium
How is this manifested?	10%–15% increase in heart rate and blood pressure

What is the advantage of rocuronium?	Rapid onset that gives adequate muscle relaxation for rapid sequence intubation in patients with a contraindication to Sch
What drugs are used to reverse NDMR?	Anticholinesterase drugs (neostigmine, edrophonium, pyridostigmine)
What drugs need to be combined with these reversal agents and why?	The anticholinergic drugs glycopyrrolate or atropine are used to counteract the profound vagal stimulation evoked by the anticholinesterases.

OPIATES

What opiates are commonly used in the ICU?	Morphine and fentanyl
What are the primary therapeutic effects of the opiates?	Analgesia and sedation
What are their effects on respiratory drive?	Decreased respiratory drive, manifested primarily as decreased respiratory rate and secondarily as decreased tidal volume
Which opiate causes the greatest histamine release?	Morphine
Which opiate is the better anxiolytic?	Morphine
Which opiate is more potent?	Fentanyl
What is the most commonly used narcotic antagonist?	Naloxone

BENZODIAZEPINES

What are the four most commonly used benzodiazepines (BZDs) in the ICU?	1. Midazolam (Versed) 2. Diazepam (Valium) 3. Lorazepam (Ativan) 4. Chlordiazepoxide (Librium)

What are the clinical effects of BZDs?	Anxiolysis, hypnosis, anticonvulsion, skeletal muscle relaxation (no analgesia!)
Which is the shortest acting BZD?	Midazolam (1.5–3.5 hrs)
How are BZDs metabolized, and why is this important?	Hepatically. Geriatric patients and patients with liver failure are likely to have prolonged duration of action.
Which BZD is traditionally used for delirium tremens prophylaxis and alcohol withdrawal?	Chlordiazepoxide (Librium)
What is the BZD antagonist?	Flumazenil (Romazicon)
Which BZD is not primarily metabolized hepatically?	Serax

MISCELLANEOUS SEDATIVE AGENTS

What is the therapeutic effect of propofol (Diprivan)?	Generalized CNS depression similar to the barbiturates, but without analgesic effects
What are the advantages of propofol over benzodiazepines or barbiturates?	1. Rapid changes in level of sedation by simply changing infusion rate 2. Rapid recovery, usually within 10–15 min, after a bolus dose or after stopping an infusion 3. Development of physical dependence does not seem to occur. 4. Also may have antiemetic properties

INOTROPIC AGENTS

DOPAMINE

Site(s) of action and effect at:	
Low dose (1–3 µg/kg/ min)?	++ dopaminergic (D_1 and D_2 receptors) receptor activation: renal and mesenteric vasodilation causes increased renal and mesenteric blood flow, respectively (so-called "renal dose dopamine").

Intermediate dose (2–5 μg/kg/min)?

+ α_1, ++ β_1 receptor activation: increased inotropy and chronotropy, as well as some vasoconstriction.

High dose (> 5 μg/kg/min)?

+++ α_1 receptor activation: marked afterload increase due to arteriolar vasoconstriction.
Dopaminergic and β-adrenergic effects are still present but usually somewhat overshadowed by α-adrenergic effects.

DOBUTAMINE (DOBUTREX)

Site(s) of action?

+++ β_1 and β_2 receptors

Effects?

1. Increased inotropy (β_1 effect)
2. Decreased afterload (β_2 effect)
3. Mildly increased chronotropy (β_1 effect) that can lead to increased myocardial oxygen demand (MVO2) and tachycardia.

Dosage?

5–15 μg/kg/min. Tolerance to dobutamine develops in about 72 hours due to downregulation and uncoupling of β-adrenergic receptors.

MILRINONE (PRIMACOR)

Mechanism of action?

Phosphodiesterase III (PDE III) inhibitor, which inhibits the breakdown of cyclic adenosine monophosphate (cAMP) and therefore increases intracellular cAMP and intracellular calcium availability

Effects?

1. Increased inotropy
2. Decreased afterload
3. Little to no increase in chronotropy, with no net increase in MVO2
4. Mild pulmonary vasodilatory effect

Dosage?

1. Load: 50–75 μg/kg over 10 minutes
2. Maintenance: 0.375–0.7 μg/kg/min

ISOPROTERONOL (ISUPREL)

Sites of action?

+++ β_1 and β_2 receptors

Effects?	1. Increased inotropy (β_1 effect) 2. Increased chronotropy (β_1 effect) 3. Vasodilation of skeletal, mesenteric, and pulmonary vascular beds (β_2 effect)
Dosage?	1. Load: 0.02–0.06 mg 2. Maintenance: 0.5–10 μg/min

EPINEPHRINE (ADRENALINE)

Sites of action?	α_1, α_2, β_1, and β_2 receptors
Effects?	1. Increased inotropy (β_1 effect) 2. Increased chronotropy (β_1 effect) 3. Not much change in blood pressure at low doses (0.04–0.1 μg/kg/min) due to peripheral vasodilation (β_2 effect) 4. Can have marked increases in blood pressure at higher doses (α_1 effect)
Dosage?	1. Load: 0.25–1 mg 2. Maintenance: 1–4 μg/min

NOREPINEPHRINE (LEVOPHED)

Sites of action?	α_1, α_2, and β_1 receptors
Effects?	1. Increased inotropy (β_1 effect) 2. Increased chronotropy (β_1 effect) 3. Marked increase in blood pressure (α_1)
Dosage?	Begin at 0.5–1 μg/min and titrate to effect up to 8–12 μg/min.

INTRAVENOUS ANTIHYPERTENSIVE AGENTS

NITROGLYCERIN (NTG)

Effects?	1. +++ venodilation (increased venous capacitance and decreased preload) 2. + arteriolar dilation 3. Inhibits platelet aggregation
Dosage?	5–100 μg/min

SODIUM NITROPRUSSIDE (NIPRIDE, SNP)

Effects?

1. +++ venodilation (decreased preload)
2. +++ arteriolar dilation (decreased afterload)
3. Balanced effects on venous and arterial tone allows for blood pressure titration.

Dosage?

0.5–10 μg/kg/min

Side effects?

1. Hypotension
2. Hypoxia due to intrapulmonary shunting
3. Cyanide toxicity with prolonged infusions (> 48 hrs; can diagnose by obtaining thiocyonate levels)

ESMOLOL (BREVIBLOC)

Site of action?

β_1-adrenergic receptor (antagonist). Very short half-life (9 minutes) necessitates continuous intravenous infusion and allows it to be easily titrated.

Indications?

1. Short-term control of ventricular response rate in patients with atrial fibrillation with rapid ventricular response or with other supraventricular tachyarrhythmias
2. Rapid control of blood pressure, often in conjunction with SNP, in patients with a hypertensive emergency or with aortic dissection

Dosage?

1. Load with 500 μg/kg/min × 1 minute; then use a maintenance infusion of 50 μg/kg/min × 4 minutes.
2. If insufficient response, repeat loading infusion for 1 minute and increase maintenance infusion to 100 μg/kg/min × 4 minutes.
3. May repeat loading dose and increase maintenance infusion rate to 200 μg/kg/min as needed.

DIURETICS

What is the most commonly used loop diuretic in the ICU?	Furosemide (Lasix)
What are its common indications?	Acute pulmonary edema, fluid overload
What are its common side effects?	1. Hypokalemic hypochloremic metabolic alkalosis 2. Sensorineural hearing loss
What is a commonly used osmotic diuretic?	Mannitol (Osmitrol)
What is its common indication?	To reduce intracranial pressure (ICP)
What is a common side effect?	Can initially cause an acute increase in intravascular volume that may precipitate pulmonary edema
What is a commonly used aldosterone antagonist?	Spironolactone (Aldactone)
What is its common indication?	Fluid overload in the setting of cirrhosis

PROPHYLACTIC AGENTS IN THE ICU

What are the indications for stress ulcer prophylaxis (SUP)?	1. Prolonged mechanical ventilation (> 48 hours) 2. Steroid therapy 3. Severe burns or trauma (some would say that any patient staying in an ICU more than 48 hours should receive SUP)
What four classes of medications can be used for SUP?	1. Antacids 2. H_2 blockers 3. Cytologic barrier (e.g., sucralfate [Carafate]) 4. H^+/K^+ pump inhibitor (e.g., omeprazole [Prilosec])

What are the four H₂ blockers in clinical use?	1. Cimetidine (Tagamet) 2. Ranitidine (Zantac) 3. Famotidine (Pepcid) 4. Nizatidine (Axid)
What two interventions are most commonly used as DVT and PE prophylaxis?	1. Sequential compression devices or Venodynes on the lower extremities 2. Subcutaneous (SQ) heparin injections (usually 5000 units SQ every 12 hours)
What is Virchow's triad of the etiology of thrombosis?	1. Stasis 2. Hypercoagulable state 3. Endothelial damage
What are the five steps in the treatment of DVT/PE?	1. Heparin bolus 5–10,000 units IV 2. Heparin infusion to maintain heparin partial thromboplastin time (PTT) at about 1.5–2 times control 3. Begin warfarin (Coumadin) therapy about 24–48 hours after PTT at therapeutic levels. 4. Anticoagulate to a PT international normalized ratio (INR) of about 2–3. 5. Maintain anticoagulation for 3 months.
What should you, as a young trainee, know about the medications that the patient is taking?	You should consider yourself to be your patient's primary physician in the ICU and you should know what drugs they are taking, the actions, possible reactions, side effects, and other issues such as half-life, interactions, etc.
What should you do if you don't know all about the pharmacology of the medications your patient is taking?	You should look it up.
What is a good reference source?	The single most reliable source of information of this sort is the Hospital Formulary Book, which is put together by the American Association of Hospital Pharmacists. This book is unbiased, has no advertising in it, and addresses all of the pertinent issues about the drugs used in the ICU.

In general, what sorts of medications should be chosen for critically ill patients?

1. Try to choose short-acting drugs. These have immediate responses and can be stopped if their effects are not beneficial for the patient.
2. Use drugs with which you are familiar. Frequently, there are many representatives of a class of drugs, and it is a good strategy to choose one with which you will become completely familiar.

Which drugs can be administered through the endotracheal tube?

Remember the mnemonic, LANE:
1. Lidocaine
2. Atropine
3. Naloxone
4. Epinephrine
(Remember, these agents must be diluted in at least 10 ml of IV fluid and administered at about 2–2.5 times the usual dose.)

5

Anesthesia in the ICU

What is the single most important principle regarding the use of anesthetic agents in the ICU?

Be certain that the side effects of the anesthetics do not cause undue risk to your patient. No one dies of acute pain, but patients die when they lose control of their airway, quit breathing, or suffer cardiac depression from the inappropriate use of some medications.

How low should your threshold be for intubating a patient in the ICU?

Extremely low. By the time you have thought about this question more than once, you have probably waited too long to intubate your patient.

What are some indications for intubation?

1. Inability of the patient to breathe spontaneously
2. Impending loss of airway due to swelling or excessive secretions
3. Obtundation
4. Respiratory rate over 40 respirations/min
5. PCO_2 greater than 60
6. PO_2 less than 60
7. Head injury
8. Acute respiratory distress syndrome (ARDS)
9. The need for general anesthesia

In the ICU, whose responsibility is it to manage the airway and to administer anesthetic medications?

The primary health care team's responsibility (not the anesthesiologist based in the operating room). This line of responsibility or authority is the same for virtually all issues in the ICU; it is no different for anesthetic issues.

Must muscle relaxants be reversed after cardiac surgery?

No. In general, by the time the patient is awake enough to be extubated after such surgery, the muscle relaxants have worn off. However, care should be taken in those patients who have severe renal or hepatic disease, as the effects of these drugs may be prolonged. And remember, muscle relaxants have NO general anesthetic properties.

How do you evaluate residual muscle paralysis after administration of a muscle relaxant?

1. Nerve stimulator: the response to train-of-four and tetanic stimulation can be assessed. (Remember, this can be extremely uncomfortable to the unanesthetized patient.)
2. The best clinical test is the patient's ability to sustain a head lift for 5 seconds. (A successful response correlates well with adequate return of pharyngeal and laryngeal protective reflexes.)

What is the most likely cause of a so-called "endotracheal tube cuff leak"?

Improper position of the endotracheal tube, not failure of the cuff itself. Proper repositioning of the tube will usually take care of the leak. The most dangerous possibility is esophageal intubation. Listen over the stomach to help assess this possibility.

When intubating the trachea, how does one determine correct tube placement?

1. Detection of end-tidal CO_2 (the most rapid and reliable indicator of proper tube placement, if this technique is available)
2. Presence of equal, bilateral breath sounds
3. Viewing humidity in the tube on exhalation
4. Absence of breath sounds over abdomen
5. Maintenance of oxygen saturation on monitor
6. Presence of adequate chest excursion on inspiration
7. Confirmation by chest x-ray
8. Good view of the vocal cords on direct laryngoscopy

What are the hemodynamic effects of sufentanil and fentanyl?

Bradycardia and reduced blood pressure due to their vagotonic effects and depression of central sympathetic drive

What hemodynamic effect does morphine cause that fentanyl and sufentanil do not?

Hypotension via histamine release

What effects do narcotics have on ventilation?

Suppression of ventilation in a dose-dependent manner. They blunt the normal response to a rise in carbon dioxide by depressing the respiratory centers in the brain stem.

Anesthesia for cardiac surgery is often based upon the administration of large doses of opiate drugs such as morphine, fentanyl, or sufentanil. Why?

Opiates provide adequate surgical analgesia with negligible direct myocardial depression when used with muscle relaxants and oxygen.

Intraoperative (or postoperative) bradycardia in cardiac surgical patients may be a symptom of what conditions?

1. Myocardial ischemia
2. Systemic hypoxia (especially true in children)
3. Sinoatrial (SA) node or atrioventricular (AV) node dysfunction (resulting from surgical manipulation of the heart or from cardioplegia, etc.)
4. Hypothermia
5. Increased vagal tone—either drug induced (fentanyl) or reflex (pain and endotracheal intubation)
6. Drugs (such as neostigmine, β-blockers, calcium-channel blockers and cardiac glycosides)
7. Intracranial hypertension (Cushing reflex)

The oxyhemoglobin dissociation curve predicts an increase in delivery of oxygen to tissues ("right shift") in response to what physiologic changes?

1. An increased $[H^+]$ (i.e., decreased blood pH)
2. Increase in PCO_2 (via the Bohr effect)
3. Increase in temperature
4. Increase in 2,3-diphosphoglycerate (DPG); use the mnemonic "RIGHT" for right shift:
   Rise
   In
   G (2,3-DPG)
   H+
   Temperature

Why are transfused red blood cells theoretically less likely to unload oxygen to tissues than the patient's own red cells?

Stored blood has the following characteristics:
1. Decreased 2,3-DPG
2. Decreased temperature
3. Decreased pH (all of which shift the oxyhemoglobin curve to the left)

Before coronary artery bypass surgery, a patient develops characteristic symptoms of angina that are accompanied by ST-segment depression on EKG. What basic interventions could one consider to improve the myocardial oxygen-supply-to-oxygen-demand ratio?

Improve supply:
1. Increase FIO_2 (nasal cannula, face mask, etc.).
2. Check hemoglobin and consider transfusion of RBCs to improve oxygen-carrying capacity.
3. Administer nitroglycerin; this dilates the coronary arteries

Decrease demand:
1. Administer nitroglycerin; in addition to dilating the coronary arteries, it decreases loading conditions of the heart.
2. Decrease the patient's anxiety with morphine.
3. Control the heart rate (β-blockers or calcium channel blockers).
4. Control the blood pressure (afterload is an important determinant of myocardial oxygen demand).
5. Consider intravascular volume overload as an inciting factor (diuretics or even phlebotomy may be considered).

Which nondepolarizing relaxants in current use do not require either hepatic metabolism or renal excretion for termination of their effect?

1. Atracurium (elimination by spontaneous Hoffman degradation in the plasma)
2. Mivacurium (metabolized by plasma cholinesterase)

Prolonged neuromuscular blockade after the administration of a nondepolarizing neuromuscular blocking drug may be caused by what conditions?

1. Hepatic or renal disease that precludes the metabolism or elimination of the drug(s)
2. Hypothermia
3. Electrolyte abnormalities, e.g., abnormal magnesium, calcium, or phosphorus
4. Undiagnosed myasthenia gravis (oculobulbar myasthenics are notorious)

5. Concomitant administration of other drugs such as aminoglycoside antibiotics or magnesium sulfate, which act to prolong the blockade

Succinylcholine, the only depolarizing neuromuscular blocker available in the U.S., can induce a life-threatening hyperkalemia if administered to what kind of patients?

1. Burn patients
2. Denervated patients such as hemiparetics, paraplegics, etc.
3. Patients with closed head injury
4. Patients with intra-abdominal infections
5. Patients with degenerative neuromuscular disease
6. Trauma patients (usually massive soft tissue trauma)

When mechanically ventilating patients, which measurable parameter is better correlated with barotrauma, peak airway pressure or mean airway pressure (platelet pressure)?

Mean airway pressure. Peak pressure reflects the resistance to airflow in the proximal airway and the ventilator circuit, whereas the mean airway pressure generally reflects pressure in the alveoli themselves, which is correlated with barotrauma.

Postoperatively, a cardiac transplant patient develops bradycardia. In addition to ensuring adequate oxygenation, you administer a dose of atropine which produces no increase in heart rate. Why is this expected in cardiac transplant patients, and what measures can be used quickly to increase heart rate?

The transplanted heart is denervated. Therefore, the transplanted SA node has no vagal input (the site of atropine's action) and would not be expected to increase the heart rate. Electrical pacing via temporary wires placed during surgery or β-adrenergic agonists, such as isoproterenol (which work on receptors in the transplanted pacemaker cells) will increase the heart rate in these patients.

When during the mechanical ventilator cycle should pressure measurements be made from a CVP or PA catheter?

At end-expiration (remember: ventilator and "valleys")

During the respiratory cycle in a spontaneously breathing patient?

At end-inspiration ("patient peaks")

6

ICU Radiology

Whose responsibility is it to interpret all films and studies done on the ICU patient?

You, the primary doctor, and your health care team have this responsibility. It is also your responsibility to review these studies with a more knowledgeable physician if you are not sure how to interpret them. However, you must not rely on the radiologist to pick up every subtlety of the patient's radiologic changes or to call you if the results are abnormal.

What is the single most important radiologic study in the ICU?

The chest x-ray

When should chest x-rays be obtained for patients in the ICU?

An x-ray is obtained daily on most ICU patients, especially if the patient is intubated and has central lines, chest tubes, and other devices in place. An x-ray should also be obtained every time the patient comes and goes from the ICU, since these devices have an uncanny way of hooking onto doorknobs and bedposts and being pulled out during movement around the hospital.

What structures need to be identified on an ICU chest x-ray?

Lines—? Correct location/heart chamber
Tubes—? Correct location
Bones—? Lytic lesions/fractures
Lungs—? Infiltrates/effusions/air
Heart—? Size/shape (e.g., water bottle = pericardial effusion)

Of what use is the ultrasound in the ICU?

Very useful for evaluating the gallbladder, kidneys, bladder, and fluid collections. Ultrasound-guided aspiration of fluid collections, especially in the pleural space, can also be very useful.

How may CT scans be used in critically ill patients?

To delineate the state of the pulmonary parenchyma, details about the pleural spaces, perfusion of various organs, fluid collections, areas where free air has collected, and the presence of contrast in various organs such as the ureters and bowel

Can a CT scan be dangerous?

Yes, because the patient must leave the safe haven of the ICU and go on a risky "road trip." This is why unstable patients should be accompanied by you or another member of the health care team.

PULMONARY RADIOGRAPHY

What is the most common chest radiographic abnormality in the ICU patient?

Atelectasis

What is atelectasis?

This is a term that is synonymous with collapse of a portion of the lung. It results when there is incomplete alveolar distension and can involve an entire lung or small peripheral pulmonary subdivisions. In the ICU setting, atelectasis is most frequent and most severe at the left lung base.

Describe the radiographic appearance of atelectasis.

With minimal atelectasis, the chest x-ray is normal. More pronounced atelectasis produces consolidation and volume loss predominantly in the bases of the lungs, obscuring the diaphragm and cardiac silhouette.

What are the most typical chest radiographic findings of left lower lobe atelectasis?

1. Loss of definition of the margin of the left hemidiaphragm and the lateral border of the descending aorta (termed "silhouetting" of the diaphragm and the descending thoracic aorta)
2. Increased density in the retrocardiac region on lateral view
3. Depression of the left hilar structures
4. Shift of the mediastinum to the left hemithorax

5. Hyperlucency to the left upper lobe as it overexpands to compensate for the collapsed left lower lobe

How is the diagnosis of pneumonia established radiographically in an ICU patient?

Radiographic findings are nonspecific, but include:
1. Nondescript infiltrates
2. Acinar shadows
3. Air bronchograms
4. Segmental consolidation and asymmetric consolidation (misdiagnosis rate is as high as ⅓ in ICU patients)

What are the characteristic chest x-ray findings of pulmonary edema?

Pulmonary edema secondary to CHF produces:
1. Hilar congestion
2. A "butterfly" configuration of increased vascular markings
3. Peribronchial cuffing
4. Cephalization
5. Kerley B lines
6. Pleural effusions (however, findings on chest x-ray can be very nonspecific, particularly in noncardiogenic pulmonary edema)

What are the radiographic features of ARDS?

1. The chest x-ray is usually normal for 12–24 hours after the initiating insult, but the latent period decreases with increasing severity of the insult.
2. Usually 24 hours after the insult, bilateral perihilar haze develops, followed by ill-defined linear opacities extending from the hilum consistent with interstitial edema.
3. By 36 hours, a diffuse, patchy pattern of alveolar edema is present.
4. Subsequently, there is little radiographic change unless complicated by pneumonia. (As with conditions previously described, radiographic features of ARDS are not specific and vary over the course of the disease process. Hence, serial radiographs are required. The chest x-ray may improve dramatically following the use of PEEP.)

What are the differential diagnoses of a patient with acute respiratory insufficiency and the radiographic appearance of a diffuse interstitial and alveolar process?

1. ARDS
2. Pulmonary edema
3. Aspiration pneumonia
4. Drug toxicity
5. Severe infection
6. Pulmonary contusion
7. Pulmonary embolism
8. Fat embolism

How do you diagnose a deep vein thrombosis (DVT)?

1. Venography is the gold standard; however, it is invasive, requires contrast and radiation, and can by itself induce venous thrombosis.
2. Real-time B-mode ultrasound is now the most commonly used modality; however, ultrasound cannot reliably detect iliac and pelvic thromboses.
3. MRI can reliably detect thrombosis of not only the femoral veins but also the pelvic veins. This option should be considered if ultrasound of the legs is negative and suspicion is high.
4. Impedance plethysmography has generally been replaced by ultrasound.

What diagnostic tests are used to confirm a pulmonary embolism (PE)?

The extent to which one needs to confirm the presence of a PE is controversial.

1. Pulmonary arteriogram; the gold standard, but invasive
2. Ventilation-perfusion scintigraphy (V/Q scan); now commonly used and results are given as low, medium, and high probability. High probability scans usually indicate a PE. However, many PEs do not result in high probability scans and, in addition, this test's accuracy goes down significantly when there are ventilation defects or an abnormal chest x-ray before the onset of symptoms of a PE.
3. Have a very low threshold for moving directly to a pulmonary arteriogram. If therapy will be altered by a positive result and clinical suspicion is high, proceed with arteriogram.

4. Normal scan with a low clinical suspicion—PE very unlikely.

What are the radiographic characteristics of traumatic pulmonary contusion?

Chest x-ray usually abnormal on admission, but abnormalities can be delayed for up to 6 hours. Areas of contusion frequently adjacent to solid structures. Opacities may appear as either homogeneous air-space consolidation or an irregular and coarse interstitial form. Resolution begins by 24–48 hours and is complete by 1 week.

What are the radiographic characteristics of fat embolism syndrome?

Chest x-ray findings are nonspecific, but usually normal early in the course. Patchy opacities subsequently develop that usually become diffuse within 72 hours. As in pulmonary edema, there is usually perihilar and basilar predominance with sparing of the apices. Clearing of the chest x-ray usually takes 7–10 days.

What are the findings of a pneumothorax on a chest radiograph?

A pneumothorax is characterized by the presence of a thin, smooth, well-defined visceral pleural line outlined by air in the pleural cavity on one side and the lung parenchyma on the other side. No pulmonary markings can be detected peripheral to this line.

What radiographic "tricks" may be used to facilitate detection of a pneumothorax?

A pneumothorax may be difficult to detect on a supine chest x-ray because the air may become loculated in an anterior location. Therefore, it is important to obtain either an upright chest x-ray or a contralateral lateral decubitus film (i.e., left lateral decubitus chest x-ray to rule out a right-sided pneumothorax) during expiration, to facilitate detection of the pneumothorax.

What is a pulmonary infiltrate?

A generic radiographic term that describes a white, poorly marginated density in the lung field that is the result of material that has permeated or infiltrated into the alveoli or adjacent tissues of the lung parenchyma. This can be secondary to an inflammatory process (infection, collagen vascular disease, allergic reaction), hemorrhage (trauma, vasculitis), proteinaceous material, cellular components (malignancy), or simple fluid (inhalation injury, drowning).

What is a pleural effusion?

Fluid within the pleural cavity. It may be simple (as seen with CHF) or complex as seen with infections (pus) or trauma (blood).

How can one determine whether a pleural effusion is free flowing?

To help determine whether the fluid in the pleural space is free flowing, a decubitus chest x-ray with the affected side dependent can be obtained. If the fluid is free flowing, there will be redistribution of the fluid to the dependent portion of the pleural cavity.

Why are pleural effusions, pneumothoraces, and free air in the abdomen often difficult to discern on films taken in the ICU?

Due to the fact that most ICU films are exposed with the patient in the supine position, abnormal gas and fluid collections do not assume their "classical" positions and configurations. For this reason, it is important to obtain either upright, lateral, or decubitus films when clinical suspicion is high to maximize the accuracy of the radiographic diagnosis.

Pulmonary edema is the term used to describe an abnormal amount of fluid in the extravascular tissues of the lung. What are some causes of pulmonary edema?

Use the mnemonic "A,B,C,D,E,F,G,H,I,J,K,L,M":
Aspiration of liquids
Brain injury/neurogenic causes
Cardiac decompensation (CHF)
Drug reaction (allergic reaction to drug)
Emboli (post-traumatic, fat emboli, PE)
Fluid overload
Gas inhalation
High altitude
Injury to the thorax
Junkie (intravenous drugs)
Kidney failure with fluid overload
Left atrial tumor obstructing pulmonary venous return
Miscellaneous (blood transfusion, rapid re-expansion of the lung, circulating

toxins such as snake venom, and
pulmonary veno-occlusive disease).

GASTROINTESTINAL RADIOGRAPHY

True or False: Inadvertent intubation of the trachea with a nasogastric or feeding tube is prevented by a cuffed endotracheal tube.

False. Tracheal intubation is possible and there may be no cuff leak. This is particularly true of feeding tubes. As a result, all tubes should have their positions verified radiographically before instilling material into them.

True or False: Patients are unable to talk if the trachea is intubated with a feeding tube.

False. Although patients may have some difficulty talking or have a weak voice, these are not reliable findings.

What markings help distinguish small and large bowel?

1. Valvulae conniventes (also called plicae circulares), which are thin, regular circumferential markings present in the small bowel; described as a "stack of coins'
2. Haustra, thick, less regular markings that are not circumferential and are present in the large bowel

What two clinical entities most commonly produce bowel distension?

Bowel obstruction and adynamic ileus

How can ileus and obstruction be differentiated on plain radiographs?

1. Ileus: in general, ileus produces generalized distension of the entire intra-abdominal portion of the GI tract, with gas present from the stomach to the rectum. Localized inflammatory processes can produce a localized ileus with short segments of distended bowel.
2. Obstruction: produces distension proximally with relative decompression distally. However, these findings can be less pronounced early in the course of obstruction or, in the case of a partial bowel obstruction, serial radiographs may be needed.

If small bowel obstruction is suggested by plain radiographs, what should be determined, if possible, about the nature of the obstruction?

Partial small bowel obstruction should be distinguished from complete obstruction and from a closed loop obstruction. Whereas partial small bowel obstruction may respond to nasogastric decompression, complete and closed loop obstruction can rapidly progress to bowel ischemia and necrosis.

What suggests the presence of partial vs. complete small bowel obstruction on plain radiographs?

Gas in the bowel distal to the area of obstruction suggests the presence of partial obstruction. However, care must be taken in interpreting this finding, as gas is present in the distal bowel early in the course of total obstruction. Hence, serial films are mandatory.

Do normal films rule out small bowel obstruction?

No. Distended loops may be filled with fluid and not be visualized on plain radiographs. Closed loop obstruction in particular may not be distended with gas and may progress rapidly to necrosis.

What other radiographic studies may be useful in the diagnosis of small bowel obstruction?

1. CT scan may be useful if closed loop obstruction is suspected.
2. Oral barium studies may be useful in selected cases when differentiation of partial vs. complete obstruction is difficult. However, oral barium should be avoided if colonic obstruction cannot be ruled out.
3. Enteroclysis can be used instead of a routine follow-through to determine the level of obstruction and may actually relieve partial small bowel obstruction due to adhesions.

With colonic dilatation, from either obstruction or ileus, what cecal diameter should raise the possibility of perforation?

When the diameter reaches 14 cm, the risk of perforation increases rapidly and decompression must be undertaken.

In colonic obstruction, what radiographic test should be performed to identify the obstruction?

Barium enema. This test should be avoided, however, if there are signs of acute inflammation or perforation.

What are the plain radiographic findings that suggest intestinal ischemia?

Findings are nonspecific but include:
1. General or localized distension
2. Thumbprinting (due to mucosal edema)
3. Bowel wall thickening
4. Pneumatosis intestinalis
5. Portal air

What radiographic tests may be used to localize GI bleeding?

Angiography, 99m Tc-labeled RBC scan, and 99m Tc sulfur colloid scan

Describe the benefits and drawbacks of each.

1. Angiography: very accurate in localizing the source and can be therapeutic. It requires a higher rate of blood loss to be positive than the tagged red cell scan.
2. 99m Tc RBC scan: can be positive at a very low rate of blood loss but many clinicians do not believe that it is specific enough in its localization of the site of bleeding. It remains in the circulation and can show active bleeding up to 24 hours after dosing.
3. 99m Tc sulfur colloid scans: can be used to localize bleeding but its excretion by the hepatobiliary system limits its usefulness.

What is the minimum rate of blood loss that angiography and tagged red cell scans are able to detect?

0.5 ml/min and 0.1 ml/min, respectively

What is the significance of free air on abdominal films and what are the best views to visualize it?

Free air suggests perforation of a hollow viscus. An upright chest film that visualizes the diaphragm and a left-side-down decubitus film are the best views to demonstrate free air.

How long can free air be visualized on abdominal films after laparotomy?

Free air is usually absorbed by 7–10 days and is rare after 14 days.

What is the initial radiographic study of choice when cholecystitis is suspected?

Ultrasound

What is the accuracy of ultrasound in the diagnosis of calculous cholecystitis?

Better than 90% accurate

What ultrasound findings are indicative of calculous cholecystitis?

1. The presence of stones in the gallbladder or biliary system
2. Sonographic Murphy's sign (pain from direct pressure of the transducer on the gallbladder)

Both 1 and 2 are very specific for cholecystitis. Other sonographic features include:

3. Gallbladder distension
4. Sludge
5. Subserosal edema
6. Intraluminal membranes or debris
7. Pericholecystic fluid

When is biliary scintigraphy (HIDA, PRIDA scans) useful in the diagnosis of cholecystitis?

In equivocal cases of calculous cholecystitis due to cystic duct obstruction (90%–95% sensitivity) or in cases of acalculous cholecystitis (lower sensitivity)

What are some causes of falsely positive biliary scintigraphy scans?

Falsely positive results may be obtained in any condition that produces stasis and distension of the gallbladder including prolonged illness, hyperalimentation, recent postoperative state, and hypoperfusion. In addition, hepatocellular dysfunction can produce false positives.

How is the diagnosis of acalculous cholecystitis established?

Although diagnosis is frequently based on clinical findings, serial sonograms demonstrating progressive changes in the gallbladder wall, especially the development of subserosal edema, are suggestive of the diagnosis. Other findings may include intraluminal membranes, asymmetric wall thickening, and pericholecystic fluid.

What is the upper limit of the normal diameter of the common bile duct?

The upper limit of normal is 7–10 mm, with most surgeons using 10 mm as the cutoff in their clinical decision making.

What is the imaging study of choice in severe pancreatitis?

Dynamic CT. Bolus intravenous contrast is given while images are taken through the pancreas. Pancreatic edema and fluid collections can be identified, as well as areas of necrosis within the pancreas.

What is the best screening radiograph to rule out free intraperitoneal air (pneumoperitoneum)?

An upright chest radiograph or a radiograph of the upper abdomen that includes both hemidiaphragms. Free air rises and will accumulate underneath the diaphragm in an upright patient. This can be visualized as a translucent collection of air limited by the thin, curvilinear density of the diaphragm. It is easier to recognize on the right side, because the air density contrasts nicely with the density of the liver. If the patient is critically ill, or otherwise unable to sit upright, a left lateral decubitus film of the upper abdomen will allow the gas to rise and be detected between the right lobe of the liver and the abdominal wall.

What is the best study to determine whether there is free intraperitoneal fluid?

An ultrasound of the abdomen and pelvis can be done portably in critically ill patients. Ultrasound is also useful for localizing fluid. A CT scan can demonstrate the presence of free intraperitoneal fluid but is more costly and requires the patient to make a trip to the radiology department.

What radiographs should be obtained when there is concern for small bowel obstruction?

Supine and upright or left lateral decubitus radiographs of the abdomen

What are the findings of small bowel obstruction on the plain radiographs of the abdomen?

1. Supine film: distended loops of small bowel arranged in a ladder-like configuration
2. Upright or decubitus film: multiple small bowel air fluid levels, with the fluid level in one end of the loop different in height from the fluid level in the other end of the loop. With a complete small bowel

obstruction, there is usually an absence of gas within the colon and rectum.

CARDIOVASCULAR RADIOGRAPHY

What percent of traffic fatalities are due to traumatic aortic dissection?

15%

What percent of patients with aortic transection survive to reach the emergency room?

15%

If untreated, what percent of initial survivors will die?

90%

What percent of patients with aortic transection have a normal chest x-ray?

~ 5%

What is the usual location of injury in traumatic transection of the aorta?

Injury is at the aortic isthmus in the vast majority of cases (site of attachment of ligamentum arteriosum).

List the findings on chest x-ray that suggest aortic transection.

Aortic injury correlates with signs of mediastinal hemorrhage. These are:
1. Widened mediastinum
2. Tracheal deviation to the right (left wall of trachea to the right of T4 spinous process)
3. Deviation of the NG tube to the right (across T4 spinous process)
4. Loss of a distinct aortic knob or the lateral wall of the descending aorta
5. Left apical cap
6. Displacement of left and right paraspinal interfaces
7. Depression of left main-stem bronchus
8. Thickening of the right paratracheal strip
9. Left hemothorax

Do isolated first and second rib fractures correlate with aortic transection?

No. Although previously thought to indicate increased risk, such fractures are no longer used as an indication for arteriography.

If aortic transection is suspected, what is the diagnostic test of choice?

Aortography

Does CT play a role in the diagnosis of aortic transection?

The role of CT is in evolution. Some authors recommend its use when the chest x-ray is negative with the appropriate mechanism of injury or when the chest x-ray is equivocal. One-centimeter continuous dynamic scans from the manubrium to the carina are recommended. Any indication of aortic injury or mediastinal hematoma by any radiographic modality is an indication for aortography, and this remains the gold standard.

What is the current study of choice to diagnose aortic dissection?

Aortography

What radiographic findings on chest x-ray suggest the presence of a pericardial effusion or pericardial tamponade?

1. The cardiac silhouette is triangular, globular, or flask-shaped.
2. Normal indentations of the cardiac border are lost.
3. Hilar shadows may be obscured.
4. Lateral chest x-ray shows encroachment of the retrosternal space.
5. The pericardial stripe is widened to greater than 2 mm.
6. Separation of the epicardial and anterior mediastinal fat planes is visible on lateral projection (reported to be the most reliable sign and present in about half of cases).

What diagnostic test may be used to confirm the presence of a pericardial effusion/tamponade?

1. Echocardiography: the preferred initial test
2. CT scan: if visualization is inadequate by echocardiography or more precise resolution is needed
3. Subxiphoid pericardial window: for unstable patients

Outline the noninvasive imaging modalities available to assess cardiac function, myocardial perfusion, and myocardial infarction.

1. Echocardiography: most frequently used modality to assess cardiac function and anatomy. Chamber size, ejection fraction, wall thickening, segmental motion abnormalities, presence of mural thrombi, presence of ventricular aneurysm, and valve motion can all be assessed and performed at bedside. However, it is user dependent, and quality can frequently be limited by body habitus.
2. MUGA (multiple-gated acquisition study): utilizes 99m Tc-labeled red cells and gated radioisotopic imaging gated to diastole and systole to assess ejection fraction, contractility, and segmental motion abnormalities
3. Myocardial perfusion imaging: utilizes thallium-201 chloride to assess perfusion of the myocardium. This isotope is treated similarly to potassium by myocardial cells and requires an intact Na^+/K^+–ATPase pump for uptake. Viable ischemic cells will demonstrate uptake after resolution of ischemia, and this provides the basis for stress thallium imaging.

When the head and neck of an adult are in the neutral position, what is the preferred location of the tip of an endotracheal tube?

Approximately 5 cm above the carina. With flexion or extension of the head and neck from a neutral position, the location of the tip of the endotracheal tube can vary by 2 cm in a caudad or cephalad position, respectively.

What is the desired position for the tip of a central venous catheter inserted from a subclavian or internal jugular vein approach?

In the superior vena cava, with the tip positioned so that it lies in a parallel course with the lateral walls of the superior vena cava. On a frontal view chest x-ray, this position would correspond to a location approximately one vertebral body caudad to the adjacent carina.

What is the desired location of the tip of a Swan-Ganz catheter for hemodynamic monitoring?

Within the right or left main pulmonary artery. A more peripheral location can lead to pulmonary infarction and a more central location could lead to cardiac arrhythmias and the inability to obtain satisfactory pulmonary capillary wedge pressures.

What is the desired location for the tip of an intra-aortic counterpulsation balloon pump?

Just caudal to the left subclavian artery. On a frontal chest x-ray, this corresponds to a location slightly cephalad to the adjacent carina.

What is the desired position for the tip of a nasogastric suction tube?

At least 10 cm caudal to the location of the gastroesophageal junction. Some of the nasogastric tubes are fenestrated and have proximal sideholes. All of the sideholes of the nasogastric tube should be positioned within the stomach. The approximate location of the gastroesophageal junction on a frontal chest x-ray is at the level of the left cardiophrenic angle.

To minimize gastroesophageal reflux and the subsequent potential for aspiration, where should the tip of the nasoenteral feeding tube be?

Within the duodenum and beyond the pyloric channel of the stomach to prevent reflux of feedings into the stomach. If the distal portion of the nasoenteral feeding tube is positioned within the third portion of the duodenum, the distal aspect of the tube will have a characteristic "C" configuration on an abdominal radiograph.

What should you do if you have any doubt about the location of the feeding tube?

You should not use it.

What findings on a chest radiograph might suggest inadvertent intubation of the esophagus rather than the trachea?

Small lung volumes and gaseous distension of the esophagus and stomach. Although the most common cause of gaseous distension of the stomach in a critically ill patient is aerophagia, gaseous distension of the stomach with or without gaseous distension of the esophagus should raise the concern for inadvertent placement of the endotracheal tube into the esophagus.

What are relative contraindications to intravascular administration of contrast during a radiographic examination?

1. Allergy to iodine or history of allergic reaction to contrast material. A history of allergy to contrast material or iodine places the patient at risk for a life-threatening reaction to intravascular contrast material. This risk can be reduced by giving the patient a steroid preparation, beginning 12 hours before the procedure and using nonionic contrast material.

2. Renal insufficiency. Patients with underlying chronic renal insufficiency are predisposed to developing contrast-induced acute renal failure. This risk can be minimized by aggressively hydrating the patient before administration of intravascular contrast.

7

Monitoring

How reliable are the monitors used in the ICU?

The reliability of these monitors is far from perfect. Their reliability is determined partly by how well they were set up initially, including how well lines and catheters are positioned and maintained. If some data do not fit with the other information available, then these data must be either disregarded or obtained in some other way to corroborate a finding that is an "outlier."

What is the purpose of hemodynamic monitoring?

To assess volume status and cardiac output

What monitoring issues could arise that would kill your patient in the next 24 hours and what can you do to lessen the likelihood of these issues arising?

1. Access misadventures. Use care in line insertion and check placement with pressure, waveform monitoring, and chest x-ray.
2. Pulmonary artery catheter-induced arrhythmias. Consider pacing catheter if left bundle branch block (LBBB) is present. Don't let PA catheter remain in RV.
3. Pulmonary artery rupture caused by PA catheter. Don't overwedge catheter; don't edge if not necessary; don't wedge while on cardiopulmonary bypass (catheter is cold and stiff); don't leave catheter sitting outside mediastinal shadow on chest x-ray.

What are some clinical indicators of perfusion in an ICU patient?

1. Urine output is probably the best clinical indicator of perfusion. A well-perfused adult patient should generally have 0.5–1 ml/kg/hr of urine output.
2. Feel the patient's feet and hands. A well-perfused patient will have warm extremities, with brisk (less than 1 second) capillary refill.

3. Normal mentation is often listed as a sign of adequate perfusion, but many patients in the ICU have been sedated, making this assessment difficult.
4. Patients with inadequate perfusion are often tachycardic.

What are the most fundamental monitoring devices for invasive and noninvasive monitoring in the ICU?

Arterial lines, central venous lines, Swan-Ganz catheters (PA catheters), BP cuffs, oxygen saturation monitors, and the end-tidal CO_2 monitor.

How reliable is an experienced physician's estimate of volume status by examination of the patient?

About as reliable as flipping a coin. Studies have shown that even very experienced physicians are hardly better than 50% accurate in assessing a patient's volume status. Thus, there is need for invasive monitoring if fluid status must be known.

In blood gas reports, the term "torr" is used in lieu of the older term, "mm Hg." What is the origin of the term "torr"?

The "torr" unit has come into use to recognize Evangelista Torricelli, an Italian physicist of the 17th century who is credited with having originated the idea of the mercury manometer.

What does a pulse oximeter measure?

Peripheral arterial blood oxygen saturation

How do the following affect the affinity of oxygen for hemoglobin?
• **Decreased pH**
• **Increased temperature**
• **Increased 2,3 DPG**
• **Increased PCO_2**

All will favor decreased oxygen affinity and increased oxygen delivery. Thus, all shift the oxygen dissociation curve to the right. (Remember the caricature of George Bush on Saturday Night Live saying "that's good, that's good" about any shift to "the right.")

What are three sources of error encountered when measuring pressures with a fluid-filled catheter (e.g., arterial line, Swan-Ganz catheter)?

1. Deterioration in frequency response. Check for air or clot in the catheter/transducer.
2. Catheter whip. As the catheter is hit by the pulse wave, motion is generated, which increases systolic

pressures and lowers diastolic
pressures; i.e., the mean pressure is
unaltered. This can also be tested in
arterial lines by inflating a BP cuff
proximal to the line; as the cuff is
deflated, the pressure that
corresponds to the first pressure wave
recorded on the arterial line is the
true systolic pressure.
3. Catheter impact, which is caused by a
valve hitting the catheter

What is the Allen's test?

It is a test used to detect adequate
collateral ulnar circulation before placing
a radial arterial line.

Is the Allen's test useful?

It has been shown that in the absence of
peripheral vascular disease, the Allen's
test is not an accurate predictor of hand
ischemia. In fact, the results may be
abnormal in approximately 3% of young,
healthy individuals.

**What are the differences
between arterial pressure
measurements taken in the
peripheral vs. central
positions?**

The mean BPs decrease as the distance
from the aortic valve increases, but
systolic pressure actually increases.

**What are some common
locations for arterial lines?**

1. Radial artery (most common, fairly
   safe)
2. Femoral artery (second most common
   site and probably the safest)
3. Brachial artery (most dangerous due
   to risk of arm ischemia)
4. Axillary artery (uncommon, but
   occasionally useful, and relatively
   safe)
5. Temporal artery (uncommon and
   unsafe)
6. Dorsalis pedis artery (uncommon and
   relatively safe)

**What are some
complications of arterial
lines?**

1. Infection (very uncommon)
2. Distal embolization (relatively
   uncommon)
3. Occlusion of the artery (more
   common in smaller arteries)

4. Bleeding. Be especially vigilant when an attempt has been made to place a line that seems as though it has been unsuccessful and then the site of attempted puncture is ignored. A patient can bleed to death from an attempt at femoral artery cannulation that may have seemed unsuccessful but that actually produced an arterial puncture.
5. Air embolism

When measuring BP invasively, at what level should the transducer be placed?

The transducer should be at the level of the left atrium.

What happens to the BP measurement if the transducer is not at heart level?

A transducer below heart level will falsely elevate the BP measurement, and a transducer placed too high will provide a falsely low measurement.

If one is unable to maintain an arterial line in a patient, what are some alternative, less invasive techniques that can give similar information to the arterial line?

1. Mechanical BP cuff that cycles on a regular basis
2. Oxygen saturation monitor
3. End-tidal volume CO_2 monitor (if the patient is intubated), which can give a very good approximation of the arterial PCO_2 (the end-tidal CO_2 is usually about 5 mm Hg lower than the arterial CO_2).

What is the pulse pressure?

(Systolic BP – diastolic BP)

What conditions are associated with a wide pulse pressure?

1. Aortic regurgitation
2. Sepsis
3. Thyrotoxicosis
4. AV fistulas
5. Any high output state

What condition is associated with a narrowed pulse pressure?

Hypovolemic shock

METHODS TO DETERMINE CARDIAC OUTPUT

What is the thermodilution (TD) method of measuring cardiac output?

Injecting a known quantity/temperature of fluid into the RA and measuring the bolus transit time

When determining cardiac output by the TD technique, what does the area under the curve represent?

The area under the curve represents the change in temperature of the injectate over time. There is an inverse relationship between the area under the curve and the output; i.e., a larger area indicates a lower output.

What are five pitfalls of this method?

1. Low outputs (outputs < 2.5 L/min average a 35% overestimation), tricuspid regurgitation
2. Improper technique (i.e., slow injection, incorrect volume)
3. Intracardiac shunts (VSD), extracardiac shunts (AV fistula)
4. Cold patients
5. Distal tip of the catheter in the main PA
6. Changes in blood viscosity (anemia or polycythemia)
7. Insertion of PA catheter is invasive.

How does the injectate volume affect the cardiac output measurement by the TD technique?

Injection of the wrong volume will produce an abnormal curve. For example, a lower volume than programmed will produce a falsely elevated cardiac output, and a larger volume will produce a falsely low measurement. The fundamental idea is that a higher cardiac output will dilute the cold injectate more than a low cardiac output. Thus, a low volume injected makes it seem as if the standard volume injected were more dilute, suggesting a higher cardiac output.

For a postoperative cardiac patient, what cardiac index indicates a severe reduction in cardiac function?

Less than 2.0 L/min/m^2

Name the five determinants of cardiac output.	1. Heart rate and rhythm 2. Preload 3. Afterload 4. Contractility 5. Compliance
What valvular lesions will produce errors in cardiac output determination?	Tricuspid and pulmonic valvular regurgitation (will falsely increase the area under the curve, providing a falsely decreased cardiac output)
Define arterial oxygen content (CaO$_2$).	Arterial oxygen content = (HgB) × 1.34 × %O$_2$ saturation + PO$_2$ × 0.003

What is the Fick equation?

A technique to estimate cardiac output when a pulmonary artery catheter is not present.
Fick Equation:

$$C.O. = \frac{VO_2}{8.5\ (CaO_2 - CvO_2)}$$

(Where C.O. = cardiac output, VO$_2$ = oxygen consumption, CaO$_2$ = arterial oxygen content, and CvO$_2$ = mixed venous oxygen content)

or

$$C.O. = \frac{125\ ml\ O_2/min/ml}{8.5\ [(1.34)(Hgb)\ SaO_2 - 1.34\ (Hgb)(SvO_2)]}$$

Name three pitfalls.	1. Intracardiac shunts 2. Oxygen consumption is difficult to measure (thus is generally estimated at 125 ml/min). 3. Incorrect data (e.g., estimated PaO$_2$ saturation vs. measured); this is a problem with some blood gas machines that estimate the saturation based on a nomogram for arterial blood.
What indicator does the Fick principle use?	Oxygen consumption

SWAN-GANZ CATHETERS

What is the ultimate indicator of volume status?	Left ventricular end-diastolic pressure (LVEDP)

What is the best means to estimate LVEDP in an ICU?	Via a Swan-Ganz catheter that estimates left-sided pressures by right heart catheterization
What is a Swan-Ganz catheter?	A pulmonary artery catheter with a balloon on the tip to allow the blood flow to carry it from the superior vena cava, through the heart, to the pulmonary artery. It has ports for pressure measurements and blood sampling from the right atrium and the pulmonary artery.
What are the indications for placement of a Swan-Ganz catheter?	1. Uncertainty over fluid status especially when either the heart or the kidneys are not working optimally 2. When right-sided cardiac pressures do not correlate with left-sided cardiac pressures (LV dysfunction, pulmonary hypertension, right heart failure, cardiac valvular dysfunction) 3. To assess left ventricular function in situations in which this function is unknown
What is the characteristic Swan-Ganz tracing in acute mitral regurgitation?	"V" wave in the wedge tracing representing regurgitant flow into the left atrium
What is the characteristic finding in acute ventricular septal rupture?	An oxygen saturation step-up in the pulmonary artery as compared with the right atrium
What Swan-Ganz tracings are suggestive of a hemodynamically significant pulmonary embolus?	Elevated right heart pressures (central venous pressure [CVP], pulmonary artery systolic [PAS], pulmonary artery diastolic [PAD]), with normal wedge pressure
What pressure profile is seen in cardiac tamponade?	Equalization of all central pressures (CVP, PAD, pulmonary capillary wedge pressure [PCWP]); high value = 30 cm H_2O).
What complications may occur with a Swan-Ganz catheter?	1. Ventricular ectopy during placement is caused by irritation of the bundle of His fibers at the RV outflow tract. Treatment consists of advancing or retracting the catheter away from this point.

2. Pulmonary artery rupture is seen when the balloon is inflated and the catheter is so peripheral that it already fills the vessel it is in and is usually caused by distal migration of the catheter or advancing it with balloon deflated. This complication may be prevented by avoiding balloon hyperinflation (less than 1.5 ml) and advancing the catheter only with the balloon inflated. The most common presenting symptom is acute hemoptysis. There is a very high mortality rate associated with this complication.

3. Pulmonary infarction can occur if the catheter balloon is inadvertently left inflated, causing ischemia to the segment of lung parenchyma supplied by the segmental artery into which the catheter has been floated.

4. Right bundle branch block during placement may cause complete heart block in the presence of preexisting left bundle branch block.

What factors predispose patients to pulmonary artery rupture with placement of a PA (Swan-Ganz) catheter?

1. Pulmonary hypertension (difficult to obtain wedge)
2. Advanced age
3. Coagulation at the catheter tip (difficult to obtain good wedge tracing)
4. Cardiac operations (catheter gets pushed in further during manipulation of the heart and becomes stiff during systemic cooling)

If the Swan-Ganz catheter does not wedge, what can be used to approximate LVEDP?

PAD pressure

When does PAD not correlate with the wedge pressure?

In severe lung disease with pulmonary vascular changes

What can be directly measured with the Swan-Ganz catheter?

1. Central venous right atrial pressure
2. Pulmonary artery pressures

3. Pulmonary capillary wedge pressure (left atrial approximation)
4. C.O. (via the thermodilution technique)
5. Mixed venous oxygen saturation

What are the clinical signs of decreased intravascular volume?

1. Mental status changes
2. Low BP
3. Tachycardia
4. Drop in urinary output
5. Dry mucous membranes
6. Poor skin turgor
7. Arterial pressure decrease with ventilator-delivered breaths.

What is the cardiac index (CI)?

C.O. divided by body surface area (BSA) in square meters; normal = 2.5 – 4 L/min/m^2

How do you calculate the systemic vascular resistance (SVR) index?

$$SVR = \frac{80\ (MAP - CVP)}{C.O.}$$

Where MAP = mean arterial pressure and CVP = central venous pressure; normal = 900 – 1400 dyne · sec · cm^{-5}). Remember Ohm's law: resistance = pressure/flow.

What is the PCWP?

The downstream pressure against the tip of the catheter once it has been "wedged" in place in the distal pulmonary artery. The wedge pressure is a reflection of the left atrial pressure and, therefore, the LVEDP (i.e., the filling pressures of the left side of the heart).

When is the PCWP not a good indicator of left heart filling pressures?

1. Mitral valve dysfunction (stenosis, regurgitation)
2. High PEEP
3. Pulmonary veno-occlusive disease

**How do PCWP, C.O., and
SVR change in the
following situations?**

Table 7–1

	PCWP	CO	SVR
Septic shock	Down	Up	Down
Hypovolemic shock	Down	Down	Up
Neurogenic shock	Down	Down	Down
Cardiogenic shock	Up	Down	Up

**How does the Swan-Ganz
catheter help to detect
early myocardial ischemia?**

Myocardial ischemia causes a decrease
in left ventricular compliance; i.e., the
ventricle becomes stiffer. Consequently,
the presence of an elevated PCWP or
the development of prominent A or V
waves on the PCWP tracing may be
early signs of ischemia.

**In which patients does a
Swan-Ganz catheter
provide more useful
information than a CVP?**

The Swan-Ganz catheter is useful in
patients who need measurements of
PCWP, C.O., and SVR. In patients with
normal ejection fractions (EF), a CVP
correlates well with the PCWP. In those
with a poor EF (less than 40%), those
with pulmonary artery hypertension, and
those with right heart failure, CVP
correlates poorly with PCWP; in such
cases a pulmonary artery catheter would
be indicated.

**A Swan-Ganz catheter is
placed via the right
subclavian vein. All
pressure measurements
are satisfactory, but the PA
pulse wave recording is
continuously dampened.
What might one find on
chest x-ray to explain this
annoying problem?**

The right angle turn at the junction of
the right subclavian vein with the
superior vena cava often produces a kink
in the Swan-Ganz catheter at this point,
producing a dampened waveform on the
monitor.

In placing a central venous line via the right subclavian vein, the guidewire and catheter seem to pass OK, but with slight resistance encountered at about the 15-cm mark on the catheter. Venous blood is easily aspirated from it, however. The patient reports pain in the region of the right ear. What malposition of the venous catheter might be noted on x-ray?

Passage of the venous line cephalad into the right internal jugular vein

How can this problem be corrected?

With the use of fluoroscopy, by trying to rewire the line, by holding pressure on the neck while advancing the wire, or most commonly, by inserting the line elsewhere.

What is the most common early complication of a central venous line insertion?

Pneumothorax

What is a potential complication of even briefly disconnecting a large-bore central venous line?

Air embolism

What rhythm disturbance may ensue if a newly placed central venous line extends into the right ventricle?

Ventricular tachycardia

When placing an internal jugular venous cannula, how can the clinician ensure proper placement in the vein and not the artery?

1. The blood returning on initial attempt with the finder needle should be dark without evidence of pulsatile flow.
2. The cannula can be transduced after ensuring good venous flow. Transducing can be accomplished either by attaching to a transducer

and monitoring the venous waveform, or by attaching a long plastic tube to the cannula and ensuring a rise and fall of the fluid column with respiration.

When a central venous line must be replaced due to suspected infection and there is no new site available, what procedure might be used?

A new catheter can be placed at the same site over a guidewire passed through the lumen of the old catheter.

What are some locations in which one can gain access to the central venous circulation?

1. Internal jugular vein (commonly used for monitoring)
2. Subclavian vein (most commonly used for parenteral alimentation)
3. Femoral vein (most commonly used in code situations or states of hypovolemia)
4. Supraclavicular subclavian vein (an uncommonly used but very reliable line)

List the potential central venous access points in order of safety during the acute phase of placement from safest to most dangerous.

1. Femoral vein
2. Supraclavicular subclavian vein
3. Internal jugular vein
4. Infraclavicular subclavian vein

Which is the only central line that should be used in states of significant hypovolemia such as trauma and code situations?

Femoral venous line

What are the functions of central venous lines?

1. Central venous pressure monitoring
2. Administration of hypertonic or vasoactive substances that cannot be administered safely in peripheral veins, such as parenteral alimentation and vasoconstrictors (dopamine)

What are some complications of central line placement?

1. Pneumothorax
2. Inadvertent arterial puncture
3. Bleeding from venous puncture sites
4. Vein thrombosis

5. Malposition of catheters
6. Infection
7. ediastinal hemorrhage from great vessel injury

What are some aids in placing central lines?

1. Know the anatomy completely and have a three-dimensional picture of the spot at which you want to enter the vein.
2. Use the Seldinger technique (small needle, guidewire, larger catheter).
3. Consider the possibility of a small seeker needle that can be left in place while the larger needle is tracked parallel to it.
4. Make liberal use of a Doppler probe to listen for venous sounds to guide your cannulation attempts.
5. Mark the skin with a marker once you have determined the anatomy by palpating landmarks, listening with the Doppler, and making a conscious effort to visualize the location of the vein.

Must every patient in an ICU have a central line and an arterial line?

No. But working on critically ill patients without these devices is usually the exception rather than the rule.

How do you avoid septic complications from central lines?

1. Follow strict sterile procedure when placing lines (broad sterile fields, mask, gown, closed glove technique, don't let J wires touch anything dirty).
2. Don't allow lines with dextrose (sugar water) in them to be violated.
3. Rewire the lines frequently (every 3 days if feasible), culture the tips, and rotate sites if these tips grow bacteria.
4. Always consider the line as a potential source when patient is becoming septic (confused, febrile, etc.).

ICU FORMULAS AND NORMAL VALUES

Oxygen consumption (VO_2)?
= (arterial oxygen content − mixed venous oxygen content) × cardiac output × 10 = (1.34 ml O_2/g Hgb × [Hgb] × (SaO_2 + 0.0031 x PaO_2) − 1.34 ml O_2/g Hgb × [Hgb] × $SmvO_2$ + 0.0031 × PaO_2) × CO × 10

Normal range of VO_2?
= 250 ml/min. (Add 13% for each degree C increase in temperature.) Remember!! Coefficients of oxygen utilization range in various vascular beds from 0.6% to 0.85% of delivered oxygen. Hence, a minimal oxygen delivery of 500 ml/min is required for a 70-kg patient with a basal oxygen consumption of 250 ml/min and an additional 50 ml/min due to stress (i.e., 300 = 0.6 × 500).

Oxygen delivery (DO_2)?
= CaO_2 (arterial oxygen content) × CO × 10 = (1.34 ml O_2/g Hgb × [Hgb] × SaO_2 + 0.0031 × PvO_2) × CO × 10

Normal range of DO_2?
= 900 − 1100 ml/min

Arteriovenous oxygen difference ($DAVO_2$)?
= CaO_2 − CvO_2 = (1.34 × [Hgb] × SaO_2 + 0.0031 × PaO_2) − 1.34 × [Hgb] + SvO_2 + 0.0031 × PvO_2)

C.O.?
$$= \frac{VO_2}{8.5\,(CaO_2 - CvO_2)} \quad \text{(Fick equation)}$$
= heart rate (HR) × stroke volume (SV) = HR × (end diastolic volume − end systolic volume)

Normal range of C.O.?
= 4–6 L/min

CI? (C.O. / BSA)
= 2.5–4.5 L/min/m^2

Mean aortic pressure (MAP)?
= diastolic BP + ⅓ (systolic BP − diastolic BP)

Normal MAP?
= 95 mm Hg

Stroke work (SW)?
= SV × MAP

SVR?	Remember Ohm's law: $V = IR$; hence, $R = V/I = \dfrac{80 \ (MAP - CVP)}{C.O.}$
Normal range of SVR?	$= 1200 \pm 300$ dyne $\cdot$ sec $\cdot$ cm^{-5}
SVRI?	$= SVR \times BSA$
Normal range of SVRI?	$= 2100 \pm 500$ dyne $\cdot$ sec $\cdot$ cm^{-5}
Pulmonary vascular resistance (PVR)?	$= 80 \times$ (mean pulmonary artery pressure - mean left atrial pressure)/ C.O.
Normal range of PVR?	$= 100 \pm 50$ dyne $\cdot$ sec $\cdot$ cm^{-5}
What is the PVRI?	PVR $\times$ BSA
What is the normal PVRI?	170 ± 70 dyne $\cdot$ sec $\cdot$ cm$^{-5} \cdot$ m^{2}
What are Wood units?	Used in heart transplant evaluations: $\dfrac{PA \ (mean) - PCWP \ (mean)}{CO \ (normal < 4)}$ Remember, the SVR, PVR, etc. are calculated numbers; i.e., errors in pressure or C.O. measurements will affect these numbers. For example, a patient with a normal C.O. of 6.0 L/min and significant tricuspid regurgitation may have a measured C.O. of 3.0 L/min. This would double the calculated SVRI and may result in inappropriate treatment.

NORMAL FILLING PRESSURES

Right atrial pressure (RA or CVP)[mean]?	$= 0$–8 mm Hg
RV pressure (systolic/ diastolic)?	$= 15$–$30/0$–8 mm Hg
PA pressure (systolic/ diastolic)?	$= 15$–$30/3$–12 mm Hg
PCWP (mean)?	$= 3$–12 mm Hg

What is the PCWP?   Approximates the left atrial and the left
                                      ventricular pressure during ventricular
                                      filling

What is the PCWP useful   Determines the volume status of the
for?   patient; i.e., PCWP > 12 = volume
                                      overloaded; PCWP < 3 = volume
                                      depleted

Section 2

Intensive Care
Considerations by
Organ System

8

Central Nervous System

What CNS issues could arise that would kill your patient in the next 24 hours, and what can you do to lessen the likelihood of these issues arising?

1. Intracranial hemorrhage. Keep blood pressure under control. Be sure patient isn't overanticoagulated. Don't infuse thrombolytics for more than 24–48 hours.
2. Herniation. Monitor pressure. Reduce cerebral edema. Prevent unnecessary straining.
3. Uncontrolled seizure activity (status epilepticus). Don't completely paralyze a patient who is seizing until seizure is controlled. Optimize antiseizure medications.
4. Hypoglycemic neurologic injury. Monitor glucose levels. Be sure to avoid reactive hypoglycemia (and run D10 if total parenteral nutrition [TPN] is stopped). Don't control glucose too tightly with insulin drip.
5. Alcohol withdrawal. Keep potassium and magnesium high. Administer thiamine, B_{12}, and folate. Consider benzodiazepine prophylaxis. Consider low-dose ETOH infusion.
6. Occult bleeding from trauma. Perform CT scan if neurologic status changes.
7. Meningitis. Maintain a low threshold for lumbar puncture if neurologic status changes in a febrile or immunosuppressed patient.
8. Hypotension. Pay attention to usual oxygen delivery issues (e.g., cardiac output, volume, arrhythmias).
9. Anoxia. Ensure that respiratory status is stable.

What are some elements of neurologic health maintenance in the ICU?	1. Minimize use of neurologically active drugs as much as possible. 2. Use alternative pain management strategies (e.g., epidurals, nonsteroidals, intrapleural local anesthetics) if feasible. 3. Maintain normal day/night cycles when possible. 4. Employ physical therapy. 5. Administer thiamine, folate, potassium, and magnesium to alcohol abusers before withdrawal is evident. These may all be given intravenously. Judicious use of benzodiazepines in such patients may be necessary. 6. Elevate head of bed slightly to decrease cerebral edema. 7. Have some idea of intracranial pressure (ICP) [level of consciousness, papilledema, CT scans, ICP monitoring, bolts] in patients at risk, such as trauma patients, patients with strokes, patients with brain metastases. 8. Make surroundings familiar and comfortable. 9. Don't discuss details of the patients' care in front of them. The patients will almost always be scared by what they hear. 10. Check for hypercalcemia. 11. Be sure patient is never hypoglycemic.
What condition is most commonly associated with spontaneous brain hemorrhage?	Hypertension
What symptoms are associated with a ruptured cerebral aneurysm?	Headache, neck stiffness, photophobia, and nausea
What is the single best test to diagnose meningitis?	Lumbar puncture (Gram stain and culture of cerebrospinal fluid [CSF])

What is the single most important study to obtain when a person has had a recent head injury and has an altered level of consciousness?	CT scan
What is the approximate incidence of focal neurologic deficits after cardiac surgical procedures?	2%
What are the risk factors for focal neurologic deficits after cardiac surgery?	1. Increased age 2. Diabetes 3. Preexisting cerebral vascular disease (especially history of a stroke) 4. Perioperative hypertension 5. Known or discovered ascending aortic atherosclerosis and calcification 6. Left ventricular mural thrombus 7. Opening of a cardiac chamber during surgery 8. Postoperative atrial fibrillation 9. Long duration of cardiopulmonary bypass
What are the mechanisms for central neurologic deficits after cardiac surgery?	1. Cerebral hypoperfusion (cerebrovascular disease or hypotension) 2. Particulate embolism (atherosclerotic debris, thrombus, platelet debris, or air)
How do you evaluate perioperative neurologic deficits?	Careful neurologic exam, CT scan with contrast. (Echocardiograms and noninvasive carotid studies may also be helpful.)
How are perioperative neurologic complications treated?	A CT scan must be obtained to rule out evidence of intracranial hemorrhage, which is very rare under these conditions. Once hemorrhage has been ruled out, heparin therapy can begin and is usually recommended. Standard measures to reduce ICP may be indicated depending on the extent of the injured tissue. Early institution of physical therapy is important.

What percentage of patients have an acute, transient change in mental status after a major operation?

Approximately 30%

What are the risk factors for postoperative delirium?

1. Older age
2. Alcoholism (recent)
3. Preoperative organic brain disease
4. Severe cardiac disease
5. Multiple associated illnesses
6. Prolonged cardiopulmonary bypass time

What are some common causes of postoperative delirium?

1. Medications (benzodiazepines and analgesics)
2. Metabolic disorders (especially uremia)
3. Alcohol withdrawal
4. Low cardiac output
5. Hypoxia
6. Sepsis
7. Recent stroke
8. Periods of marginal cerebral blood flow, either during cardiopulmonary bypass or anesthesia, or in the postoperative period

How is postoperative delirium managed?

1. Metabolic abnormalities must be corrected and psychoactive medications must be withheld.
2. Haloperidol 2–5 mg IV q 6 hours is a reasonable choice of therapy if alcohol withdrawal is not suspected because haloperidol reduces the seizure threshold in addition to being a tranquilizer.
3. To treat suspected alcohol withdrawal, benzodiazepines can be used but it must be remembered that they are cardiac depressants. Thiamine and folate should also be administered to chronic alcoholics.
4. It is very important to keep potassium and magnesium at the high end of normal in these patients.
5. Psychotherapy is very important and should consist of reassurance and

support from the team and from the family. The more that can be done to familiarize the surroundings, the better off the patient will be.

What are the primary types of stroke?

1. Ischemic (thrombotic or embolic)
2. Hemorrhagic (intracerebral hemorrhage and subarachnoid hemorrhage)

What are the usual locations in the brain of the various types of stroke?

1. Embolic—peripheral or cortical
2. Intracerebral hemorrhage—deep (basal ganglia, thalamus, cerebellum)
3. Large vessel thrombosis—variable, depending on the vessel
4. Lacunar infarct—pons, internal capsule (usually from hypertension)
5. Subarachnoid hemorrhage—vessels are ruptured at their junctions in the circle of Willis.

How are the different types of strokes treated?

1. Cardiac embolic stroke: first heparin, then warfarin anticoagulation
2. Cerebrovascular stroke: antiplatelet agents and carotid endarterectomy
3. Hemorrhagic stroke: lower markedly elevated blood pressure to normal range. *Caution:* overcorrection can lead to catastrophic results, especially in the situations of thrombosis and embolism.
4. Increased intracranial pressure: monitoring with ICP bolts, evacuation of clot, and even craniectomy have been used to reduce ICP.
5. Subarachnoid hemorrhage: when possible, surgical ligation or clipping of the aneurysm and antifibrinolytic agents have been used. Calcium channel blockers have also been used to reduce cerebral arterial spasm.

What is the term for transient loss of consciousness due to trauma without demonstrable anatomic change in the brain?

A concussion

What is cerebral autoregulation?

A mechanism to keep cerebral blood flow fairly constant between a mean arterial pressure (MAP) range of 50–150 mm Hg

How is it mediated?

By myogenic factors (i.e., response to changes in smooth muscle tension in vessel wall)

What is normal ICP?

5–10 mm Hg (as reflected by 70–135 mm CSF)

How is intracranial hypertension defined?

ICP greater than 20 mm Hg (with an associated CSF pressure of 270 mm)

What are signs of increased ICP?

1. Headache
2. Nausea, vomiting
3. Mental status changes
4. Cushing's reflex (systemic hypertension and bradycardia)
5. Papilledema
6. Signs of brain herniation (dilated and nonreactive pupils, unilateral motor weakness/hemiplegia)

What is the treatment for increased ICP?

1. Bed elevatation of at least 30 degrees
2. Hyperventilation (PCO_2 in low 30s)
3. Hyperosmolar agents (mannitol)
4. Steroids (for tumors)
5. Barbiturate coma
6. Craniectomy in selected cases
7. Diligent ICP monitoring via placement of an ICP bolt

What is the normal rate of cerebral blood flow (CBF) in adults?

50 ml/100 g/min

What is the effect of hyperventilation on ICP?

Decreases it.

By what mechanism?

It decreases CBF. (Chemoreceptors in the cerebral circulation cause vasoconstriction in response to decreased PO_2 and increased pH.)

By how much?	CBF decreases 2%–4% with a 1 mm Hg decrease of PCO_2.
How should a patient with increased ICP be positioned?	30-degree head elevation decreases the ICP by enhancing venous drainage from the head.
How does mannitol work to reduce ICP?	As an osmotic diuretic, it draws free water from the brain.
What are the first lines of therapy to treat increased ICP?	1. Supplemental oxygen 2. Hyperventilation 3. Mannitol (0.25–1.0 g/kg)
What does positive end-expiratory pressure (PEEP) do to ICP?	It increases ICP by impairing venous drainage from the head.
What is the effect of barbiturates on the brain?	They decrease cerebral metabolic rate by up to 60%.
What is a barbiturate coma?	Pharmacologically induced minimal electrical brain activity
What is the #1 cause of mortality after a carotid endarterectomy (CEA)?	A myocardial infarction
Causes of stridor after a CEA?	Injury to recurrent laryngeal nerve or hematoma compressing airway
What is the risk of stroke immediately after a CEA?	3%–5%
Do intraoperative shunts decrease stroke rate?	No
What is "triple H" therapy?	1. Hypertension 2. Hypervolemia 3. Hemodilution
When is it used?	To treat cerebral vasospasm after subarachnoid hemorrhage
Which group of drugs may also be used to minimize cerebral vasospasm?	Calcium channel blockers

What is "Cushing's triad"?
1. Increased ICP
2. Hypertension
3. Bradycardia

Why are severe head trauma patients given phenytoin (Dilantin)?
Posttraumatic seizure prophylaxis

What is the incidence of posttraumatic seizures?
20%–30%

What is the role of steroids in acute spinal cord trauma?
High-dose steroid therapy within the first 24 hours improves neurologic outcome.

What is the recommended steroid regimen?
30 mg/kg methylprednisolone (Solu-Medrol) during the first hour after injury, then 5.4 mg/kg/hr for 23 hours

Which vessels form the circle of Willis?
Anterior cerebral, anterior communicating, middle cerebral, posterior communicating, and posterior cerebral artery

What factors determine CBF?
$$CBF = \frac{(MAP - ICP)}{CVR}$$
where MAP = mean arterial pressure; ICP = intracranial pressure; CVR = cerebrovascular resistance

Injury of which vessels most commonly causes epidural hematomas?
Middle meningeal arteries

Injury of which vessels causes subdural hematomas?
Cortical bridging veins

Where are intracranial aneurysms most commonly located?
Middle cerebral artery

Which cranial nerves traverse the cavernous sinus?
Cranial nerves III, IV, V, VI

What is the effect of hypothermia on brain metabolism?

It decreases it.

By how much?

A 1° C decrease in temperature lowers metabolic rate by 7%.

What are some causes of altered mental status in the ICU?

Use the mnemonic VITAMIN D:

Vascular: anoxic-ischemic encephalopathy, stroke (embolic, thrombotic, hemorrhagic, fat embolus, disseminated intravascular coagulation [DIC])

Infectious: bacterial or fungal meningitis, viral encephalitis

Traumatic: diffuse axonal injury, subdural hematomas

Affective: depression, pseudocoma

Metabolic: hypoglycemia, hypercalcemia, hypercapnia, metabolic alkalosis, thyroid disorders, adrenal crisis, uremia, hepatic encephalopathy, hypothermia, Wernicke's encephalopathy

Inflammatory: aseptic meningitis, vasculitis

Neoplastic: metastases, primary CNS tumor, paraneoplastic limbic encephalitis

Drugs

What are causes of generalized weakness in the ICU setting?

Use the mnemonic MUSCLES:

Medications (neuromuscular blockers, steroids)

Unrecognized neuromuscular disease (Guillain-Barré, myasthenia)

Spinal cord injury (trauma, stroke)

Critical illness (polyneuropathy)

Loss of muscle (disuse, rhabdomyolysis)

Electrolytes (hypermagnesemia, hypophosphatemia)

Systemic diseases (diabetic neuropathy, vasculitis)

What is Guillain-Barré syndrome (GBS)?

Subacute (acute) inflammatory polyneuropathy

What features are required for the diagnosis of GBS?

1. Progressive symmetrical weakness
2. Areflexia
3. Absence of other causes of subacute

neuropathy: toxins, diphtheria, porphyria

What laboratory data support the diagnosis?

1. CSF (via lumbar puncture): elevated protein, few cells
2. EMG: consistent with demyelinating polyneuropathy

What are some complications of GBS?

1. Ventilatory failure
2. Aspiration
3. Labile blood pressure
4. Cardiac arrhythmias
5. Deep venous thrombosis (DVT)

How is GBS treated?

1. Physical therapy
2. DVT prophylaxis
3. Ventilatory support as needed
4. Early plasmapheresis (*not* steroids)

What is brain death?

Irreversible loss of all brain function (See *Ethics* chapter)

Criteria?

1. Unresponsive coma
2. Absence of brain-stem reflexes
3. Absence of reversible causes
4. Apnea

What are some causes of seizures in the ICU?

1. Prior seizure disorder (may be exacerbated by fever, sleep deprivation, drugs)
2. Posttraumatic reaction
3. Drug withdrawal, including alcohol
4. Metabolic abnormalities
5. Drug toxicity
6. Focal brain disease (stroke, tumor, abscess, viral encephalitis)

What is status epilepticus?

Repeated seizures without full recovery of consciousness between seizures

What is the treatment of status epilepticus?

1. Lab tests (CBC, chemistries)
2. Glucose and thiamine
3. Benzodiazepines: Lorazepam (4–8 mg) or Diazepam (10–20 mg)
4. Phenytoin 20 mg/kg slowly, then infusion of less than 50 mg/min IV
5. Reassessment and possible intubation
6. Second-line anticonvulsant: phenobarbital (5–10 mg/kg) or

midazolam (0.2 mg/kg), infusion
7. Pentobarbital coma (Beware of the potential for unrecognized status epilepticus in paralyzed ICU patients receiving neuromuscular blocking agents!)

What measures should you take when caring for a patient with cerebral metastases?

1. Antiseizure medications
2. Steroids
3. Avoidance of increases in ICP (e.g., keep CO_2 down, avoid straining, elevate head)

9

Respiratory System

What are some respiratory health maintenance issues for patients in the ICU?

1. Avoid aspiration—it's deadly.
2. Suction the main airway with catheters and scopes prn.
3. Keep FIO_2 < 50% (avoids oxygen toxicity).
4. Elevate the head of the bed.
5. Make sure that one half of the patient's calories comes from fat (more favorable respiratory quotient).
6. Check chest x-ray personally every day.
7. Keep airways suctioned. Consider "toilet" bronchoscopy.
8. Sample secretions for Gram stain and culture frequently.
9. Consider "physiologic" positive end-expiratory pressure (PEEP) if intubated (prevents alveolar collapse).
10. Never use a T-piece (promotes atelectasis).
11. Avoid fluid overload. (Dry lungs are healthy lungs.)
12. Employ physical therapy (e.g., chest percussion, turn patient frequently, cough).
13. Keep airway sterile (e.g., use sheathed suction catheters, sterilized bronchoscopes).
14. Check the position and function of all tubes daily (most have some relationship to lungs), including chest tubes, endotracheal tubes (ETs), and nasogastric (NG) tubes.

What respiratory issues could arise in the next 24 hours that could kill your patient, and what can you do to lessen the likelihood of these issues arising?

1. Loss of airway. Intubate patient sooner rather than later. Be sure tubes are secure. Make sure patient can't bite tube. Ensure optimal large airway toilet (frequent suctioning, toilet bronchoscopy, consider mucolytics).
2. Pulmonary edema. Maximize cardiac status. Use diuretics and manage fluid status to keep lungs dry. Intubate if necessary.
3. Virulent pneumonia. Monitor cultures. Treat virulent organisms aggressively.
4. Pulmonary embolism (PE). Deep vein thrombosis (DVT) prophylaxis. Aggressive heparinization and diagnostic workup if PE is suspected. Consider inferior vena cava (IVC) filter if PE is suspected in a patient already on anticoagulation or if high-risk patient has a contraindication to anticoagulation.
5. Aspiration. Keep GI tract decompressed. Don't rely on cuffed tubes for protection. Keep head up at least somewhat.
6. Pneumothorax. Scrutinize chest x-rays daily. Obtain chest x-ray after invasive procedures and tube placement. Ensure chest tubes are working properly. Obtain additional chest x-rays for all acute changes in pulmonary status. Minimize assaults on the thorax by inexperienced team members with needles.

What are the two basic functions of the lungs?

1. Gas exchange
2. Blood filtering

What are the indications for a chest x-ray in the ICU?

1. Any invasive procedure, such as intubation, central line placement, chest tube insertion, and thoracentesis
2. Any time a ventilated patient is moved from one bed to the next, or from one unit to another (to ensure

continued appropriate tube placement)
3. Any significant change in patient status
4. Any patient with an ET, chest tube, or pulmonary artery catheter in place should have a daily chest x-ray if one has not been obtained for other reasons.

To which level can a therapeutic bronchoscope see?

An average bronchoscope has an outer diameter of 5 mm. It is not capable of visualizing below the level of the segmental bronchi.

What are the different types of cells found lining the lower respiratory tree?

1. Type I pneumocyte (predominant): a squamous cell involved in gas exchange. It cannot reproduce.
2. Type II pneumocyte: a stem cell capable of producing new alveolar epithelial cells. It also produces surfactant but does not participate in gas exchange.
3. Clara cell: nonciliated epithelial cells found in the terminal bronchioles. Function is unknown.
4. lveolar macrophage: the scavengers that remove debris from the air spaces. They are the most common type of cell recovered in bronchoalveolar lavage.
5. Mast cells: found throughout the airways. They participate in immunologic processes.

What is total lung capacity (TLC)?

TLC is the volume of gas contained within the lung at maximal inspiration.

What is vital capacity (VC)?

VC is the greatest volume that can be exhaled after maximal inspiration.

What is residual volume (RV)?

RV is the gas remaining in the lung after maximal exhalation (VC + RV = TLC).

What is functional residual capacity (FRC)?

FRC is the volume of air that remains in the lung after a *normal* exhalation. Therefore, it is a greater volume than the RV. The difference between FRC and RV is known as the expiratory reserve volume (ERV).

What is surfactant?

Surfactant is a phospholipid secreted by type II pneumocytes of the alveolus.

Why is it important?

It lowers the surface tension, which is greatest at smaller alveolar volumes. It improves lung compliance, making it easier to inflate.

How is reflex bronchial constriction mediated?

Vagal afferents are stimulated by many different stimuli that can cause reflex bronchial smooth muscle constriction. These stimuli include instrumentation (i.e., laryngoscopy), foreign body, cold air, chemicals, gastric acid, histamine, certain prostaglandins, and leukotrienes.

How many circulations does the lung possess?

Two
1. The bronchial circulation (derived from the systemic circulation) comprises 0.5%–2.0% of the cardiac output providing nutrients to all the airways proximal to the terminal bronchioles. These vessels can proliferate and may be the major blood supply to scar tissue and tumors.
2. The pulmonary circulation is a low-pressure system that contains 10%–20% of total blood volume. It receives the entire cardiac output at low pressures as it is a low-resistance circuit.

How does acid–base status affect pulmonary vascular resistance?

Acidosis causes pulmonary vasoconstriction, and alkalosis causes pulmonary vasodilation. Both respiratory and metabolic causes of acidosis and alkalosis will have these effects.

What other factors affect pulmonary vascular resistance (PVR)?

1. PVR declines with increasing pulmonary vascular pressures by expanding the vascular bed through recruitment of additional vessels and by distension of existing open vessels.
2. PVR declines with increasing lung volumes except at very high lung volumes where capillary stretch increases resistance.

3. Parasympathetic input via acetylcholine is a weak vasodilator. Activators of β-adrenergic receptors result in vasodilatation. Norepinephrine and epinephrine mediate vasoconstriction through α-adrenergic receptors. Other vasodilators include bradykinin, prostaglandin E_1 (PGE_1), and prostacyclin. Other vasoconstrictors include histamine, serotonin, thromboxane A_2, prostaglandin F (PGF), and PGE.

4. Alveolar PO_2 is a potent regulator of pulmonary vascular tone. Arteries constrict in areas of alveolar hypoxia, resulting in a redistribution of pulmonary blood flow toward oxygen-rich areas.

TO REVIEW

What increases and what decreases PVR?

1. Hypoxia?   1. Increases

2. Hypocarbia?   2. Decreases

3. Hypercarbia?   3. Increases

4. Acidosis?   4. Increases

5. α-adrenergic stimulation?   5. Increases

6. Large tidal volumes? 6. Increases

MECHANICAL VENTILATION

What are the indications for intubation and mechanical ventilation?

Inability to maintain a patent airway, inability to prevent aspiration of secretions, inadequate alveolar ventilation ($PCO_2 > 50$), inadequate oxygenation ($PO_2 < 60$, O_2 Sat $< 85\%$) to induce a respiratory alkalosis for the management of increased intracranial pressure.

What monitors should be used during mechanical ventilation?	1. Continuous pulse oximetry 2. End-tidal CO_2 3. Arterial line for arterial blood gas (ABG) access 4. Pulmonary artery catheter for PEEP > 15 cm H_2O, especially for decreased left ventricular (LV) function, unknown fluid status, mixed venous blood gas monitoring
What are complications of mechanical ventilation?	1. Barotrauma 2. Oxygen toxicity 3. Secretion accumulation 4. Nosocomial infections (pneumonia) 5. Laryngotracheal stenosis 6. Atrophy of respiratory musculature
What is the difference between ventilation and oxygenation?	Ventilation refers to removal of CO_2 from the alveoli ($PaCO_2$), whereas oxygenation refers to delivery of oxygen to red blood cells (RBCs) [PaO_2].
What size ET is routinely used in adults?	A 7-mm diameter tube in women; an 8-mm diameter in men
Who should perform endotracheal intubation in an urgent setting?	The most experienced person available
How is proper intubation confirmed?	1. Auscultation over chest and stomach 2. Chest movement 3. End-tidal CO_2 4. Chest x-ray verification
What is the greatest danger of endotracheal intubation?	Unrecognized esophageal intubation
What should always be ordered after intubation?	A chest x-ray
What conditions may cause wheezing?	Bronchospasm, aspiration, pulmonary edema, pulmonary embolus, pneumothorax, endobronchial intubation

What are the common modes of weaning patients from a ventilator?

1. Intermittent mandatory ventilation (IMV) supplemented by pressure support
2. Intermittent periods of T-piece ventilation

What is a pressure-cycled ventilator?

Delivers set airway pressure to patient; the volume delivered depends on lung compliance.

What is a volume-cycled ventilator?

Delivers set tidal volume to patient; the pressure attained depends on lung compliance.

How is pulmonary compliance calculated?

Compliance = $\Delta V/\Delta P$, where V = lung volume (L); P = pulmonary pressure (cm H_2O)

What is physiologic dead space?

The volume of inspired air not participating in gas exchange. It is composed of the anatomic dead space (the volume of air remaining within the conducting airways at the end of inspiration) and the alveolar dead space (the amount of air within underperfused alveoli).

How can dead space ventilation be calculated?

$Vd/Vt = (PaCO_2 - PeCO_2)/PaCO_2$, where Vd/Vt = ratio of dead space to tidal volume; $PaCO_2$ = arterial PCO_2; $PeCO_2$ = exhaled PCO_2). The ratio (usually less than 0.4) is often associated with failure to wean from ventilatory support when greater than 0.6.

What is the P_{50} of hemoglobin?

27 mm Hg. It reflects the partial pressure of oxygen when 50% of hemoglobin is saturated with O_2.

What is the most common cause of respiratory alkalosis in the ICU?

Iatrogenic hyperventilation

What are the common causes of metabolic alkalosis?

NG suction, loop diuretics, antacids, volume contraction, hypokalemia, blood products, lactate administration, H_2 blockers

What are the two most important endogenous buffering systems in the body?	Bicarbonate carbonic acid system and hemoglobin
How fast does P_{CO_2} rise in an apneic patient?	6 mm Hg in the first minute, then 3 mm Hg/min
How much of the total energy is spent on the work of breathing?	1%–2% in the resting person with healthy lungs
What is described by the respiratory quotient (RQ)?	The ratio of the rate of CO_2 production to the rate of O_2 consumption $RQ = CO_2$ production $/ VO_2$
What is a normal value?	0.8 in a healthy person on a normal diet
Why measure RQ when patients are difficult to wean from ventilatory support?	Large carbohydrate loads in the nutritionally supported patient can lead to lipogenesis and increased CO_2 production. This may increase RQ to 1.0 or even greater and prevent effective weaning from ventilatory support. Increasing the percentage of calories provided as fats can reduce CO_2 production.
What blood gas parameter primarily reflects alveolar ventilation?	The Pa_{CO_2} (partial pressure of carbon dioxide in arterial blood)
Name two methods of increasing the alveolar ventilation of a patient on a volume respirator.	1. Increase the rate of ventilation 2. Increase the tidal volume
Your patient acutely develops inadequate alveolar ventilation despite correct ventilator settings. What causes must you rapidly rule out?	Remember: LIFE **L**ung: mucous plugging of bronchus, pneumothorax **I**nternal tubing: dislodgement of ET , right main-stem intubation, plugging of tube **F**ight: agitated patient fighting ventilator **E**xternal tubing: disconnection of ventilator from patient, kinking of tubing, patient biting ET

How is tidal volume defined?	The volume of air inspired during a single, regular breath
How does one determine the appropriate tidal volume for a specific patient?	10–15 ml/kg of patient's ideal body weight (IBW)
What is minute ventilation?	(Tidal volume) × (rate of ventilation)
What is FIO_2?	The fraction of the inspired gas mixture comprised of oxygen
What is the FIO_2 of room air?	21%
What blood parameters reflect the patient's oxygenation status?	The PaO_2 and the oxygen saturation
What changes in the ventilatory settings can the physician make to increase the amount of oxygen delivered to the patient?	1. Increase the FIO_2 2. Increase the PEEP
What is PEEP?	Positive end-expiratory pressure
What is "physiologic PEEP"?	3–5 mm Hg of "physiologic PEEP" exists in the normal (nonintubated) airway. Placement of an ET tube across the glottis removes this PEEP.
What does PEEP do?	PEEP holds alveolar sacs open and moves fluid out of the alveolus and into the interstitium. Oxygenation may be enhanced as PEEP increases.
How much PEEP is usually required?	Most intubated patients should have at least 5 mm Hg PEEP to replace physiologic PEEP. However, 10, 15, or even 20 mm Hg PEEP may be required by hypoxic patients with acute lung disease to achieve adequate oxygenation.

What problems are associated with high PEEP?

These high pressures can cause barotrauma in the form of subcutaneous emphysema, and bleb formation, pneumothorax, and tension pneumothorax. Further, venous return to the heart is impaired as peak airway pressure increases, causing decreased cardiac output and hypotension.

At what levels of PEEP may the cardiac output be depressed?

Patients with normal hearts will tolerate 10–15 cm H_2O of PEEP without difficulty. Patients with sick hearts may tolerate levels of PEEP above physiologic range very poorly. In patients with the most compromised hearts, even 5 cm H_2O of physiologic PEEP may make the difference between a stable low output state and frank cardiogenic shock.

What is the IMV mode?

IMV = intermittent mandatory ventilation. In this mode, the physician inputs the desired tidal volume and rate with which this volume will be mechanically delivered to the patient. The patient need not contribute in any way to the process. However, the patient may take additional breaths above the set rate, but *without* help from the ventilator. This may be difficult and uncomfortable for the patient because of high resistance in the tubing (the snorkel phenomenon) and poorly timed machine breaths that may interrupt the patient's own breathing pattern.

What is the SIMV mode?

SIMV = synchronized intermittent mandatory ventilation. Similar to IMV, except that the ventilator senses the patient's spontaneous breathing pattern and attempts to time machine-delivered breaths with the patient's breathing cycle. Spontaneous breaths remain unassisted (less fighting, but no relief from the "snorkel" effect).

What is the theoretical advantage of SIMV over IMV?

Prevents "breath stacking" (superimposing a mechanical inhalation or exhalation on spontaneous breathing, with resulting increased airway pressures). Some studies have shown that breath stacking is not a real problem. In fact, virtually all patients can be managed with the IMV mode, and it is much cheaper than SIMV.

What is the AC mode?

AC = assist-control mode. The physician inputs the tidal volume and rate, as with IMV and SIMV. However, the machine senses any patient-generated respiratory effort and immediately follows with a full, machine-powered breath. Thus, the patient does no work even to carry out his own spontaneous breaths (no snorkel problem).

What are the drawbacks of AC mode?

The machine may deliver more breaths/min than the set rate specifies, and it is hard to know how much support the patient is actually receiving. In addition, respiratory alkalosis may become a problem.

What is CMV?

CMV = controlled mechanical ventilation. It delivers a preselected ventilatory rate, tidal volume, and inspiratory flow rate independent of patient effort. However, it does not allow the patient to initiate any spontaneous breaths.

What are some indications for CMV?

1. Apnea secondary to CNS depression (brain and spinal cord trauma)
2. Drug overdose
3. Neuromuscular paralysis
(It is appropriate for the patient who is unable to initiate spontaneous breaths. It can be agonizing to the patient who attempts to ventilate spontaneously.)

What is CPPV?

CPPV = continuous positive-pressure ventilation. It is CMV with PEEP.

What is AMV?

AMV = assisted mechanical ventilation (patient-triggered positive-pressure ventilation). The ventilator will not deliver a mechanical breath without a patient-initiated breathing effort.

For what can it be used?   Weaning from CMV and promoting spontaneous breathing

What is a major weakness of AMV?   Apnea can be fatal. Also, this mode makes following the patient's improvement difficult.

What is CPAP?   CPAP = continuous positive airway pressure. It is PEEP applied during spontaneous inspiration and may be administered with or without mechanical ventilation (as opposed to PEEP, which can only be applied with a ventilator).

What is the benefit?   Increased expiratory transpulmonary pressure and lung volume (increased functional reserve capacity). This pressure is intended to keep alveoli open and lung compliance optimal.

What is pressure support ventilation (PSV)?   PSV senses the initiation of the patient's spontaneous breath and delivers a specified amount of pressure support during that breath. The beauty of this system is that the amount of pressure can be varied (usually 5–20 cm H_2O). At the higher levels, the work of breathing is very low and thus the patient's ventilation is almost fully supported by the ventilator. One warning with this ventilatory mode is that an apneic patient will get no breaths at all.

For what is PSV used?   To decrease the work of spontaneous inspiratory breathing between IMV breaths. This mode is a very useful adjunct to the IMV mode when weaning a chronic ventilator patient.

What is pressure control (PC) mode?   PC is fundamentally different from the volume-based modes: IMV, SIMV, and AC. In PC mode, the physician inputs the desired peak airway *pressure* to be delivered to the patient and the frequency with which this pressure is to be applied. The effective tidal volume, then, varies depending on the compliance or stiffness of the lungs. The benefit: a theoretical decrease in the likelihood of barotrauma in patients with very stiff lungs. The drawback: vigilant monitoring of the effective tidal volume is essential since an abrupt decrease in pulmonary compliance can decrease the minute ventilation and cause a rapid rise in P_{CO_2}.

What is mandatory minute volume?

A preset minute volume will be guaranteed through spontaneous ventilation with additional mechanical positive pressure breaths being provided by the ventilator if needed.

What is a potential drawback?

A tachypneic patient with a small tidal volume (Vt) can have inadequate alveolar ventilation without triggering mechanical assistance.

What is V/Q mismatch?

The normal pulmonary vascular bed constricts in response to local alveolar hypoxia so that unventilated alveoli receive minimal blood flow. Blood flow ("Q") is thus "matched" to ventilation ("V"). Significant regional abnormalities in blood flow (i.e., PE) or ventilation (e.g., infiltrate, contusion, effusion, pneumothorax) may overwhelm local autoregulation, causing a V/Q mismatch and resultant hypoxemia.

Can drugs cause a V/Q mismatch?

Yes! Any pulmonary artery vasodilator such as sodium nitroprusside, nitroglycerin, or nifedipine can interrupt the ability of the lung arterioles to constrict in response to hypoxia. You will see this physiology in action at the bedside! This phenomenon may exacerbate hypoxia by increasing perfusion to unoxygenated areas of the lung, which is known as shunting.

What is HPV?

HPV stands for hypoxic pulmonary vasoconstriction, and it is a response of the pulmonary vasculature to alveolar hypoxia. Oxygenation is maintained by diverting blood flow to well-ventilated areas of the lung.

What effect do pulmonary vasodilators have on HPV?

In general, all vasodilators will inhibit HPV, with the potential to exacerbate hypoxia, because unoxygenated areas of the lung will be perfused.

What five important components determine the peak inspiratory pressure (PIP) obtained during mechanical ventilation?

1. Lung-thorax compliance
2. Airway resistance
3. Delivered tidal volume
4. Inspiratory flow rate
5. End-expiratory pressure

What are typical ventilator settings?

1. Tidal volume: (Vt) 10–15 ml/kg IBW
2. Rate: 10 (8–16)
3. Mode: IMV, pressure support, etc.
4. FIO_2 (O_2 concentration): initially 100%, then ideally < 50% to prevent oxygen toxicity. Maintain hemoglobin saturation of greater than 90%.
5. PEEP: 5 cm H_2O, with 2- to 3-cm increments until Hgb saturation of greater than 90% at FIO_2 of less than 50% (avoiding cardiovascular compromise)
6. I/E (inspiratory/expiratory ratio): 1:2–3

At what levels will oxygen toxicity occur?

Oxygen toxicity may occur when the FIO_2 is greater than 50%–60% for more than 24 hours in patients with normal lungs. FIO_2 greater than 50 is potentially damaging to the lungs of critically ill patients. However, 100% oxygen for short periods of time is usually well tolerated.

What are some useful weaning parameters?

1. Resolution of original problem
2. Vital capacity (VC) > 10–15 ml/kg
3. Functional expiratory volume > 10 ml/kg
4. Negative inspiratory pressure > 20 cm H_2O
5. Resting minute ventilation < 10 L/min
6. Respiratory rate < 30/min
7. pH 7.33–7.48
8. PO_2 > 70 mm Hg on FIO_2 40%
9. PCO_2 < 50 mm Hg

Why is early weaning from mechanical ventilation preferred?

To prevent atrophy of the respiratory muscles and to minimize complications of mechanical ventilation

How is weaning done?

The rate of weaning obviously depends on the patient's strength, duration of ventilation, and other underlying conditions, such as chronic obstructive pulmonary disease (COPD). Frequently, "trial and error" by changing parameters and evaluating patient response is required. For example: decrease FIO_2 to < 50%; decrease rate (typically IMV); decrease PEEP in 2- to 3-cm increments with 6 hours between changes.

What are some causes of weaning failure?

Premature attempt to wean is most frequent. Some reversible causes: oversedation, bronchospasm, excessive secretions, acid–base imbalances, hypophosphatemia, hypothyroidism, hypomagnesemia, and hypocalcemia.

When weaning a patient from long-term ventilatory support, you must optimize all aspects of respiratory function. What considerations should there be at each of the following anatomic levels?

1. Main airway

1. Ensure efficient airway (shorten ET, maximize the size of ET, consider tracheostomy, manage large airway secretions with mucolytics, frequent suctioning, toilet bronchoscopy).

2. Smaller airways (bronchioles)

2. Bronchodilators (consider when expiratory phase is prolonged or with history of COPD, asthma, or cystic fibrosis).

3. Alveoli

3. Keep the alveoli clear and open. Reduce pulmonary edema, treat infection, consider exogenous surfactant replacement, make use of postural drainage and physical therapy such as incentive spirometry. Consider intermittent sighs or slight increases in PEEP.

4. Interstitial space	4. Reduce pulmonary edema. Treat interstitial causes of low compliance such as rejection in the setting of lung transplantation. Treat autoimmune disorders such as vasculitis with immunosuppressive agents when appropriate.
5. Pleural space	5. Evacuate fluid (transudates, pus, blood) and air from the pleural space. Make liberal use of chest x-rays, ultrasound-guided aspirations, and CT scans to plan this therapy.
6. Chest wall	6. Improve compliance to the chest wall by decreasing pain, removing restrictive dressings, keeping the patient sitting up when feasible, enhancing nutrition, and increasing strength of respiratory muscles. Treat the patient like an athlete who will condition these muscles daily.
7. Diaphragm	7. Enhance strength and mobility of diaphragm. Reduce intra-abdominal pressure as much as feasible (NG tube drainage of stomach). Consider draining ascites and re-exploring an abdomen with hemoperitoneum.
8. Other total body considerations	8. Improve overall comfort and employ psychotherapy, physical therapy, and respiratory therapy. Ensure proper amount of caloric intake from fat to enhance the respiratory quotient. Minimize additional insults to the lungs (DVT prophylaxis, assiduous protection from aspiration, control of septic foci).
What are the two most common respiratory disasters in an ICU?	1. Loss of an airway 2. Aspiration
What are the most common causes of hypoxia in the ICU?	1. Atelectasis 2. Pulmonary edema

What is the lower level of PO$_2$ that is acceptable?

60–70 mm Hg

What is an acceptable range for PCO$_2$?

30–40 mm Hg

What should one do if the PO$_2$ is low?

1. With atelectasis: suctioning, PEEP, increased tidal volume, incentive spirometer if extubated
2. With pulmonary edema: increase cardiac output, diuretics, dialysis, and sometimes add PEEP
3. Increasing the FIO$_2$ will not be effective if shunting is the cause of hypoxia, but it should be tried transiently while other treatments are being instituted.

How accurate are the designations of FIO$_2$ of the various face masks (40%, 60%, 100%)?

It is impossible to deliver reliably more than 50% oxygen except by ET (thus, oxygen toxicity is not a risk unless the patient is intubated). Don't forget, however, that in chronic CO$_2$ retainers, suppression of hypoxic drive can occur with a face mask.

What is meant by absorption atelectasis?

The nitrogen in room air acts as a stent to keep alveoli open. The more oxygen there is in the inspired mixture, the more the nitrogen stent is diminished; thus, atelectasis can occur as oxygen is rapidly absorbed. Oxygenation will usually deteriorate seemingly paradoxically. This is a further argument against using higher levels of FIO$_2$ to increase PO$_2$.

What is subcutaneous emphysema?

It's the bubbly sensation on palpation that can occur when a pneumothorax decompresses itself into the soft tissues.

Is it dangerous?

No, but it should alert the clinician to the possibility of a dangerous underlying condition such as pneumothorax or proximal airway injury. It can also occur in the setting of a chest tube or tracheostomy when air dissects into subcutaneous tissue planes around the tubes.

What is the treatment for this condition?

Better evacuation of air from the chest. Occasionally, subcutaneous emphysema is seen when there is an air leak from the bronchial tree into the mediastinum (i.e., pneumomediastinum). This can occur in the setting of injury to the bronchus itself.

Could air dissect into the pericardium and cause a tamponade effect?

This condition has been reported, but it is extraordinarily rare. Still, if deterioration in cardiac function is felt to be occurring on this basis, total decompression can be carried out by performing an anterior cervical incision analagous to what would be used for a tracheostomy without entering the trachea. This dissection will vent all mediastinal tissue planes of their air.

What are the components of treatment of acute bronchospasm?

1. Oxygen administration
2. Diuresis (especially in setting of poor cardiac function)
3. Steroids (hydrocortisone 100 mg IV q 8 × 48 hr). Short courses of steroids will not lead to increased infectious complications.
4. Inhaled bronchodilators. Almost all of these inhaled bronchodilators can be instilled into the humidifier of a ventilator so they can be given continuously.
5. β-agonists. Terbutaline given SQ can be useful, particularly in the cardiac patient. Intravenous epinephrine or isoproterenol may also be useful in this setting.
6. IV theophylline. These preparations are not good choices in cardiac patients because they are arrhythmogenic.
7. Mechanical ventilation. Have a low threshold for intubating a patient under these conditions and initiating positive pressure ventilation. This mechanical ventilatory support will provide time for instituting other therapeutic modalities.

What effect does positive pressure ventilation have on hemodynamics?

Positive pressure ventilation causes a rise in intrathoracic pressure, which may decrease venous return, causing a subsequent fall in cardiac output and blood pressure.
25–30 cm H_2O

What are the potential complications of high airway pressures?

1. Barotrauma
2. Decreased cardiac output

How can high airway pressures cause barotrauma?

High airway pressures are seen in settings of low lung compliance. Increased pressure is required to achieve equal alveolar ventilation in comparison to conditions of normal lung compliance.

How can high airway pressures lead to decreased cardiac output and hypotension?

The high positive pressure is referred to all intrathoracic structures including the great veins, reducing venous return of blood to the heart.

At what PIP does barotrauma become a significant risk?

At PIP less than 50 cm H_2O, barotrauma rarely occurs. At PIP of 50–70 cm H_2O, there is an 8% incidence of barotrauma and the incidence increases to 43% with PIP greater than 70 cm H_2O.

In general, what should be the initial ventilator settings during an acute deterioration in patient status?

- FIO_2 = 100% (Obtain blood gases frequently and wean the O_2 to maintain an SaO_2 greater than 95% and a PO_2 of at least 70 while minimizing O_2 toxicity)
- IMV mode with a respiratory rate between 12–14 breaths per minute
- Tidal volume of 12–15 ml/kg = about 700 ml for most adults
- PEEP of 5 cm H_2O

A patient with known severe COPD, if treated with supplemental oxygen, may experience impaired breathing and increasing CO_2 retention. What is the physiologic impairment that explains this phenomenon?

The patient's respiratory center in the brain is no longer sensitive to rising CO_2, since in COPD CO_2 is chronically elevated. The patient's breathing is driven by hypoxia alone and, if excessive supplemental oxygen is supplied, breathing is no longer driven at a satisfactory rate.

A patient just intubated and placed on a ventilator has no breath sounds on the left side. What is the most likely explanation?

ET extending into the right main-stem bronchus and occluding the left main-stem bronchus.

A sudden large arterial hemorrhage occurs around a cuffed tracheotomy tube that has been in place for 3 weeks. What event has most likely occurred?

Tracheoinnominate artery fistula. The inflatable cuff on the tracheotomy tube, or the tube itself, has eroded through the anterior tracheal wall and into the innominate artery.

How should this catastrophe be handled?

If possible, the patient should be reintubated through the mouth (before removing the ET) and digital pressure should be applied through the trach site to compress the innominate artery against the back of the sternum. Alternatively, an ET tube could be inserted directly through the tracheotomy stoma. A sternotomy will be required to repair this disastrous situation.

A large air leak suddenly develops in an underwater seal draining a chest tube. What event has likely occurred to cause this?

The tube may have slipped part way out with one of the several drainage holes of the chest tube outside of the chest.

A few hours after a tracheotomy is done on a respirator patient, the trach tube is accidentally dislodged from its opening. A long suture is seen extending 4 or 5 inches out of the upper end of the tracheotomy wound. For what reason did the surgeon place this suture at the time of the original tracheotomy?

To be used in a circumstance such as the one just described. The suture has been placed through the tracheal ring just above the tracheotomy incision and is extremely useful in the early postoperative period should ET dislodgement occur. The suture will allow the trachea to be lifted to the surface of the tracheotomy wound, facilitating the replacement of the airway.

What if the ET cannot be replaced immediately?

The patient should be reintubated through the mouth or some other form of airway established.

In urgent airway access, what easily palpable structure in the midline of the neck allows quick surgical placement of a tracheotomy tube?

The cricothyroid membrane, which is located between the thyroid cartilage above and the cricoid cartilage below. This area is very superficial and no important vascular structures are interposed between the skin and this membrane. Remember, there are no structures in the anterior midline of the neck that will cause patients to bleed to death faster than they will die from loss of airway.

Describe the physiologic state of the patient with this blood gas: pH = 7.24; PO_2 = 80; PCO_2 = 61; HCO_3 = 25; O_2 Sat = 92%, base excess of 0.

This patient has a pure respiratory acidosis.

What clinical scenarios might cause this?

1. Inadequate respiratory drive (oversedation, head injury)
2. Inability to maintain work of breathing
3. Airway obstruction (foreign body, blood, mucous plug, bronchospasm)

Describe the physiologic state of this patient: pH = 7.56; PO_2 = 100; PCO_2 = 20; HCO_3 = 24; O_2 Sat = 99%, base excess of –1.

This patient has an uncompensated respiratory alkalosis.

What clinical scenarios might cause this?

Hyperventilation from pain, fear, head injury or certain brain tumors, psychogenic causes

Describe the physiologic state of this patient: pH = 7.35; PO_2 = 120; PCO_2 = 65; HCO_3 = 35; O_2 Sat 98%, base excess: +8.

This patient has a compensated metabolic acidosis.

What underlying conditions would cause this?

Remember the mnemonic SLUMPEDD:
Salicylate toxicity (aspirin overdose)
Lactic acidosis (from shock, liver disease)
Uremia
Methanol intoxication

Paraldehyde intoxication
Ethylene glycol poisoning (antifreeze)
DKA (diabetic ketoacidosis) and
Diarrhea

Describe the physiologic state of this patient: pH = 7.58; PO_2 = 130; PCO_2 = 40; HCO_3 = 35; O_2 Sat: 99%, base excess +15.

This patient has a pure metabolic alkalosis.

Causes?

Excessive loss of gastric acid (vomiting, nasogastric suction), severe dehydration (contraction alkalosis), ingestion of alkaline substances (milk-alkali syndrome)

HEMOPTYSIS

What is hemoptysis?

Blood in the sputum

What is "massive hemoptysis"?

More than 600 ml of blood produced in 24 hours

Causes of hemoptysis?

1. Infection (pneumonia, tuberculosis, bronchiectasis)
2. Malignancy
3. Instrumentation (e.g., bronchoscopic biopsy)
4. Trauma

What are the treatment priorities in massive hemoptysis?

People die of asphyxiation in massive hemoptysis, not from exsanguination.
1. Maintaining adequate gas exchange is paramount. Thus, the patient should be intubated.
2. Correct any hemostatic abnormalities.
3. Localize the site of bleeding, if possible, by bronchoscopic examination during the bleeding episode. (Rigid bronchoscopy will often be required because of the need for massive endobronchial suctioning. Flexible bronchoscopy is often sufficient, however.
4. Two treatment options are available when operative intervention is not feasible or desired: selected bronchial occlusion or bronchial artery embolization.

ASPIRATION

What are some patient-related factors in the ICU that predispose a patient to aspirate?	Altered sensorium, impaired swallowing or cough, slowed gastric emptying, paralytic ileus, poorly functioning NG tube, hiatal hernia
What are some iatrogenic factors that predispose a patient to aspiration?	Premature extubation of patients, failure to reintubate patients, and feeding before the return of bowel function are common causes of aspiration in the ICU.
How can one lessen the likelihood of aspiration?	Aspiration of GI contents is a deadly, sometimes insidious process. One must be sure that the stomach does not distend with feeding. Check physical exam, chest x-rays, gastric residuals, and mental status frequently. Keep the head of the bed elevated.

Treatment of aspiration pneumonitis?

1. Immediate treatment: bronchoscopy, pulmonary toilet, cultures, eliminate cause.
2. Next stage of treatment: pulmonary toilet, consider intubation, monitor ABGs, chest x-ray. Cultures of sputum and blood are monitored for evidence of superimposed bacterial or fungal infection. Prophylactic antibiotics and steroids are helpful. The best treatment is prevention.

What are two ways aspiration can occur?

1. Antegrade (from the upper aerodigestive tract)
2. Retrograde (from the GI tract)

What are some general factors that can contribute to antegrade aspiration?

1. Neurologic impairment
2. Intubation (vocal cord dysfunction)
3. Poor cough
4. Oral, pharyngeal, laryngeal cancers
5. Tracheostomy/ventilator

What are some general factors that can contribute to retrograde aspiration?

1. Gastroesophageal reflux
2. NG tubes
3. Esophageal motility disorders
4. Gastroparesis
5. Esophageal obstruction
6. Diverticula
7. Tracheoesophageal fistula

8. Impairment of vagus nerves
   (intrathoracic surgery, especially
   pulmonary resections)

What are some complications of aspiration?

1. Upper airway colonization
2. Bronchospasm
3. Tracheobronchitis
4. Pneumonia
5. Adult respiratory distress syndrome (ARDS)
6. Death (Mendelson's syndrome)

CHEST TUBES

What are the main indications for placing a chest tube?

Evacuation of air and/or fluid from the pleural space

What anatomic landmarks are used for most chest tube insertions?

The fourth intercostal space (nipple level), anterior axillary line

Why not place the tube more inferiorly?

Risk of intra-abdominal injury, as the diaphragm can rise to the fourth or fifth interspace during expiration

Where should the local anesthetic be injected?

Skin, subcutaneous tissue, periosteum, pleura (especially the pleura)

After entering the chest with a Kelly clamp, what is the one most important step before tube insertion?

Exploring with the index finger to ensure that the lung is free from the chest wall

What size tube should one use to drain air, serous effusion, and blood, respectively?

1. Pneumothorax: 22 or 24 French (smaller tube more comfortable)
2. Pleural effusion: 28 French
3. Hemothorax: 32 French (clotting blood may clog smaller tubes)

What is the simplest drainage system?

The Heimlich valve, a unidirectional valve that simply connects to the chest tube, allowing only egress of air or fluid

Name the three chambers in a standard chest tube collection device.

Chamber 1: for fluid collection
Chamber 2: for water seal
Chamber 3: for suction control

Indications from the collection device that the tube is clotted?	Absence of respiratory fluctuation in the water seal column
How may suction be regulated?	By increasing or decreasing the level of water in the suction control chamber (i.e., varying the water level from 10 to 25 cm H_2O). Increasing the level of wall suction will only produce noisier bubbling in the suction chamber.
Does increasing the amount of bubbling in the suction chamber increase the effectiveness of suction?	No! It only makes the environment noisier.
Should a chest tube be clamped for patient transport?	Never! Clamping a tube in a patient with an air leak may lead to a tension pneumothorax. Tube should be on water seal during transport.
How should a chest tube be removed?	There is probably no difference between pulling the tube at end-inspiration or at end-expiration. The tube should be pulled quickly and sharply. Furthermore, as the tube is removed, the tract must immediately be sealed by a Vaseline gauze dressing or by tightening a previously placed purse-string stitch.

PNEUMOTHORAX

What is a pneumothorax?	It is defined as the presence of air or gas in the pleural space.
What is the pleural space?	The area between the visceral and parietal pleura. The pleural space is a potential space that contains just a small amount of lubricating fluid and that under normal circumstances does not contain air or gas.
What are common causes of pneumothorax in the ICU patient?	1. Barotrauma, secondary to high ventilator pressures 2. Central line insertion resulting in lung injury 3. Air spaces can be left in the chest after cardiac, pulmonary, esophageal,

chest wall, or intrathoracic aortic surgery.

4. Pneumothorax can also occur during tracheostomy placement.

How is a pneumothorax diagnosed?

Almost always by chest x-ray. Physical exam will frequently show decreased breath sounds and hyperresonance to percussion on the ipsilateral side.

What is a tension pneumothorax?

A collection of air in the pleural space with a pressure greater than atmospheric pressure. The increased intrathoracic pressure can lead to hemodynamic changes and cardiovascular compromise. This condition can kill a patient quickly. Thus the diagnosis must be made quickly, sometimes without a chest x-ray.

What is the treatment for a tension pneumothorax?

The immediate treatment when suspected in a patient who is severely compromised is decompression of the chest with a large-bore needle in the second intercostal space in the midclavicular line, unless a chest tube can be placed immediately.

Why are patients on ventilators at greater risk for a tension pneumothorax?

They are on positive pressure ventilation. The spontaneously breathing patient has negative pressure in the thorax. Air can be forced into the pleural space with positive pressure ventilation and is trapped there because of a ball valve–like effect. This phenomenon can create high pressures in the pleural space.

Why does tension pneumothorax cause hemodynamic compromise?

Tension pneumothorax causes impairment of venous return to the heart secondary to increased pressure in the thoracic cavity.

What is the implication of an air leak after a chest tube is placed?

The lung or bronchus has an opening that allows air to escape from the lung or bronchial tree into the pleural space and out through the chest tube. However, one must rule out an improperly positioned tube or a faulty connection outside of the chest.

What characteristics are seen in a chest tube suction apparatus when a patient has a parenchymal air leak versus a bronchial leak?	The parenchymal leaks are typically smaller and less voluminous. In rare situations, parenchymal leaks can be very large. The bronchial air leaks are more often continuous and higher volume.
Can a patient with a chest tube in the pleural space develop a pneumothorax?	Yes. The chest tube may be in a loculated space or the tube may be clogged.

PLEURAL EFFUSION

What is a pleural effusion?	A collection of fluid in the pleural space
What are some of the causes for the development of pleural fluid in an ICU patient?	Heart failure, fluid overload, pancreatitis, "sympathetic" effusions caused by intra-abdominal processes, and central line infusing fluid into the pleural space
How are pleural effusions categorized?	Exudates and transudates
What are the characteristics of an exudate?	Pleural effusion with a protein content greater than 3 g/dl and specific gravity greater than 1.016. Exudates generally reflect disease of the pleura or pleural lymphatics and include effusions related to malignancy, infectious processes, pulmonary infarction, trauma, and pancreatitis.
What are the characteristics of a transudate?	Usually are low in protein content and reflect abnormal formation or absorption of pleural fluid, as in congestive heart failure, cirrhosis, and postpericardiotomy syndrome. More recently, pleural fluid-to-serum ratios of lactate dehydrogenase (LDH) and protein have been used to differentiate transudates from exudates (pleural-to-serum LDH ratio > 0.6 and protein ratio > 0.5 is considered exudative).

Why categorize pleural effusions into these two categories?	Exudates often require aggressive treatment of the pleural space such as chest tubes or even decortication. Transudates will usually respond to thoracentesis and treatment of the underlying cause.
What is the name of a pleural effusion associated with pneumonia?	This is called a parapneumonic effusion. These effusions are sometimes sterile; when they contain bacteria, they often progress to an empyema.
How is a pleural effusion drained in an ICU patient?	By insertion of a catheter (chest tube or pigtail) or by thoracentesis. Thoracentesis is best for patients whose fluid is thin or in whom the effusion is unlikely to reaccumulate. Chest tubes are better when the fluid is thick or infected and when the patient is on a ventilator.
What are the indications for drainage of pleural fluid?	To make a diagnosis, to allow more efficient ventilation, or to prevent "trapped lung" in the case of hemothorax or empyema
What should one suspect when a large pleural effusion is present in the hours after central line insertion?	Hemothorax (vascular injury) or IV fluids (catheter in the pleural space)
What is the treatment of this pleural effusion?	Insertion of a chest tube for drainage of blood or fluid from the pleural space

PULMONARY EDEMA

What is pulmonary edema?	Accumulation of fluid in the interstitial and air spaces of the lung
What are the two general categories of pulmonary edema?	1. Cardiogenic (hemodynamic): results from increased hydrostatic pulmonary capillary pressure as in fluid overload or left heart failure (ischemia, cardiomyopathy, valvular disease) 2. Noncardiogenic: secondary to either altered permeability of the capillary membrane (sepsis, ARDS) or to decreased plasma oncotic pressure (nephrotic syndrome)

What are the chest x-ray findings in pulmonary edema?

Increased vascularity and "cephalization" (visible vascular markings in the cephalad lung fields) occur early. Kerley's B lines at the costophrenic angles imply interstitial fluid accumulation. "Bat wing" or centrally distributed opacity indicates pronounced alveolar fluid deposition. Cardiomegaly may be noted and suggests a cardiac cause of the edema.

Initial treatment of pulmonary edema?

Oxygen and diuresis with a loop diuretic should supplement treatment of underlying cause. Mechanical ventilation with addition of 5–10 cm H_2O of PEEP is very useful for severe edema. Ultrafiltration or hemodialysis is sometimes necessary for patients unable to excrete fluids readily.

How does furosemide work?

Two mechanisms:
1. Immediate venodilation after IV injection often produces rapid clinical improvement even before diuresis ensues.
2. Inhibition of chloride and sodium reabsorption in the ascending limb of Henle's loop enhances urine output.

What is the maintenance treatment for pulmonary edema?

Ultrafiltration or hemodialysis is sometimes necessary for patients unable to excrete fluids readily (e.g., renal failure). Identify and treat precipitating factors (ionotropic therapy or afterload reduction for cases of severe left ventricular failure). Mnemonic for remembering treatments for pulmonary edema: "MOSTDAMP"
Morphine (mild sedation)
Oxygen (consider intubation)
Sitting upright (alleviates orthopnea)
Tourniquets, rotating
Digoxin (improve cardiac function)
Aminophylline (optimize lung function)
Mercurials (loop diuretics)
Phlebotomy (*not* an outmoded technique)

ARDS

What is ARDS?	Adult respiratory distress syndrome
What causes it?	The condition is poorly understood. However, after severe traumatic injury or sepsis, the injured alveolocapillary membrane allows both inflammatory cells and protein-rich fluid to enter the interstitium and alveoli. The capillary–endothelial barrier is further damaged by inflammatory cells and their mediators, contributing to the large V/Q mismatch.
What are its three primary features?	1. Severe hypoxemia, refractory to increased inspired oxygen concentration 2. Diffuse pulmonary infiltrates (interstitial and alveolar) 3. Low lung compliance
What conditions can precipitate ARDS?	Sepsis, multiple trauma, shock, aspiration, multiple blood transfusions, disseminated intravascular coagulopathy (DIC), pancreatitis, fat embolism syndrome, and cardiopulmonary bypass
Describe the radiographic finding of ARDS.	Diffuse or patchy bilateral infiltrates, initially interstitia, which will rapidly progress to become alveolar. The costophenic angles are usually spared. Later, the infiltrates may take on a patchy or nodular pattern. If the patient improves, the chest x-ray will slowly return to normal. If the condition progresses, a pattern of diffuse interstitial fibrosis may occur.
How can you differentiate between cardiogenic pulmonary edema and ARDS on chest x-ray?	Generally, with ARDS you will not see pulmonary vascular redistribution, pleural effusion, or cardiomegaly.
How can the impact of ARDS on the patient be lessened?	You must treat the underlying condition! Supportive measures must be taken, which almost always include mechanical ventilation and adequate oxygenation. Fluids are managed with the goal of

maintaining the lowest possible pulmonary capillary wedge pressure (PCWP) compatible with adequate cardiac output. The overall constant goal is to maximize oxygen delivery.

What is the mortality rate of ARDS?

Greater than 50%. When accompanied by sepsis, mortality approaches 90%!

What is the most common cause of death in patients with ARDs?

Nonpulmonary multiple organ system failure

PULMONARY EMBOLISM

What is a PE?

Thrombus formed in the peripheral venous circulation, primarily the deep veins of the pelvis and thigh, that breaks free and travels to the lung where it becomes wedged in the pulmonary vascular tree

Where do most thrombi form?

The large vein of the pelvis and thigh are the origin of most clinically important PEs. Upper extremities can rarely produce emboli.

What factors in the ICU predispose a patient to a PE?

Immobility, surgery (particularly orthopedic), malignancy, pregnancy, history of smoking or using oral estrogens

What are preventive measures?

Mobility (if possible), sequential compression devices, low-dose heparin, and low-dose Coumadin are all used in patients at risk. It is currently felt that the low-dose heparin should be titrated to "bump" the partial thromboplastin time (PTT).

What symptoms might a patient report?

Pleuritic chest pain, difficulty breathing, easy fatigability, cough, hemoptysis. Patients may report pain or swelling in a leg. Most commonly they are asymptomatic. Many patients with PEs report sensing a "feeling of doom."

Physical findings?	These vary according to the severity. Mild-to-severe respiratory distress may be noted. Patients may be cyanotic, with hypotension. (Some patients present in cardiac arrest from a large embolus.) Sinus tachycardia is common.
How is the diagnosis confirmed?	Arterial blood gas studies show hypoxia and hypocarbia. A V/Q scan can be used; however, the gold standard is the pulmonary arteriogram.
How likely is a patient to have had a pulmonary embolism if the PO$_2$ is relatively normal?	Acute pulmonary embolism is extraordinarily unlikely if the arterial PO$_2$ is above 60.
What happens to the central pressures during massive acute pulmonary embolism?	The central venous pressure and pulmonary artery systolic pressure should increase acutely and markedly, especially if there is cardiovascular compromise.
What treatment do most patients with pulmonary embolism require?	The overwhelming majority of patients with pulmonary embolism are adequately treated with intravenous heparin only. The heparin will not only terminate the cycles of clot formation, but will also reduce the release of vasoactive amines that cause widespread pulmonary vasoconstriction.
What are the indications for emergency surgical pulmonary embolectomy?	1. Refractory hemodynamic compromise 2. Severe hypoxia despite mechanical intubation and ventilation 3. Continued deterioration despite anticoagulation with heparin or thrombolytic therapy
What is the most common presentation of PE?	Most PEs are relatively asymptomatic. Tachycardia, sudden-onset dyspnea, tachypnea, and low-grade fever may be signs present in some patients. The most frequent symptoms include pleuritic chest pain, dyspnea, and cough.

What are some other subtle manifestations of PE in the ICU patient?	1. Worsening hypoxemia and respiratory alkalosis in a spontaneously ventilating patient 2. Unexplained fever, atelectasis, or pulmonary infiltrate 3. Sudden onset of pulmonary hypertension and/or elevation in central venous pressure in a monitored patient 4. Unexplained tachycardia or tachypnea 5. Worsening hypoxemia, hypercapnea, and respiratory acidosis in a sedated patient on mechanical ventilation
What are the usual findings on lung exam?	The lung exam is usually normal, although there may be focal wheezing, a pleural friction rub, or rales.
What is the most common EKG finding?	Sinus tachycardia
What are the "classic" EKG findings?	A deep S-wave in lead I, prominent Q-wave in lead III, an inverted T-wave in lead III, and right axis deviation. These findings are associated with moderate-to-severe PE.
What are the most common radiographic findings on chest x-ray?	Very often the chest x-ray will be normal or unchanged. Nonspecific findings include atelectasis, infiltrates, pleural effusion, and elevated hemidiaphragm.
What is Hampton's hump?	A pleural-based, rounded ("wedge-shaped") density once thought to be specific for PE but recently shown to be neither sensitive nor specific.
What is Westermark's sign?	Another radiographic finding once thought to be pathognomonic for PE, characterized as regional oligemia, with proximal vascular fullness. This finding was also shown to be neither sensitive nor specific.
Does everyone suspected of having a PE need a pulmonary angiogram?	No. If clinical suspicion is low with normal physical exam, normal ultrasound of lower extremities looking for venous thrombosis, and "low probability" ventilation–perfusion lung scan, a

pulmonary angiogram is not mandatory. However, a very low threshold should be maintained for obtaining this safe and accurate test.

What are some of the treatment modalities for acute PE?

1. IV heparin (acute treatment)
2. Thrombolytic therapy
3. Coumadin (long-term prophylaxis)
4. Vena cava filter (for recurrent emboli during anticoagulation therapy or when a patient has a contraindication to anticoagulation)
5. Pulmonary embolectomy (last option for massive PE)

10

Cardiovascular System

What are some elements of cardiovascular health maintenance in the ICU?

1. Keep a close eye on fluid status. Most patients are relatively fluid-overloaded unless they have had recent losses (bleeding, bowel obstruction, sepsis, pancreatitis).
2. Review the rhythm and try to work toward the closest approximation of sinus rhythm at a rate of 90 that you can attain.
3. Review medications and eliminate as many cardiac depressants as feasible (i.e., antiarrhythmics, anticonvulsants, benzodiazepines).
4. Be sure that potassium and magnesium are on the high side of the normal range, and if not, replace them until they are.
5. Consider gentle enhancing of cardiac function with low-dose dobutamine or dopamine (5 μg/kg/min).
6. Review electrocardiographic (ECG) and rhythm strips daily to keep up with electrical state of the heart.
7. Remember that ICU patients are by definition not very stable. Thus, conditions that were appropriate for the heart yesterday may not be appropriate today.
8. Be sure you have instant access to the venous circulation at all times in case some cardiac event occurs suddenly.
9. Consider keeping defibrillator pads on the patient if you've seen some ventricular tachycardia or if the patient has required defibrillation.
10. Be sure blood pressure is controlled with a proper regimen.

What cardiovascular issues could arise that would kill your patient in the next 24 hours, and what can you do to lessen the likelihood of these issues arising?

1. **Arrhythmias**

1. Keep patient monitored.
Attach to defibrillator pads if at risk.
Keep potassium and magnesium on high side.
Don't let central lines or pulmonary catheters sit in RV.
Consider antiarrhythmics if arrhythmias are prevalent.
Prevent and treat alkalosis.

2. **Tamponade**

2. Be sure bleeding is controlled.
Ensure that mediastinal tubes are working if present.
Echo if effusion is suspected.
Consider possibility of tamponade after heart surgery, uremia, cancer.

3. **Cardiac ischemia**

3. Anti-ischemic agents (calcium channel blockers, nitrates)
Anticoagulants (aspirin, heparin if unstable)
Adequate oxygen delivery

4. **Declining cardiac function**

4. Monitor with cardiac output, mixed venous O_2.
Have low threshold for inotropes.
Consider intra-aortic balloon pump (IABP).
Intervene if cardiac index (CI) is less than 2.0.

5. **Aortic stenosis present**

5. No vasodilators
No hypovolemia

CARDIAC ARREST

What are the most helpful drugs in an arrest situation?

1. Epinephrine (but don't give the whole syringe at once; titrate to effect)
2. Bicarbonate
3. Calcium

How should you prepare to handle cardiac arrests?

1. Read about resuscitation.
2. Take advanced cardiac life support classes.

What are some common causes of "near" cardiac arrest?

1. Relatively rapid drop in resistance (bolus of vasodilator, rapid warming)
2. Relatively rapid fluid loss (bleeding is most common)
3. Change in heart rhythm (atrial fibrillation is common)

What should your first moves be when confronted with a patient whose BP seems to be about 60?

1. Confirm that BP is low (feel femoral pulse, flush A-line, check cuff pressure).
2. Evaluate heart rate and rhythm and treat accordingly.
3. Give calcium chloride via a central line (which buys time to evaluate further).

What is the top priority in an arrest situation?

Ventilation (which can be with a mask; it does not have to be via endotracheal tube at first)

What is a priority of almost equal importance?

Chest compression if there is no palpable pulse at any location

How should the chest of an arrest patient who has just had cardiac surgery be managed?

Usually it should be opened. However, don't perform closed chest massage on a patient with a prosthetic mitral valve, because it may be pushed out the back of the heart.

Once adequate ventilation and circulation are restored, what should you do next?

Think. You now have time to gather your wits, along with information about the patient, and begin treatment.

What are some of the steps you should follow to diagnose arrhythmias?

1. Think about the patient and history.
2. Rhythm strips are not as helpful as you might hope.
3. ECGs are good for evaluation of P waves, width of QRS, and rate.

I. BRADYARRHYTHMIAS AND HEART BLOCK

Sinus Bradycardia

What is sinus bradycardia?

Sinus bradycardia is sinus rhythm with rate less than 60 per minute.

When are patients with bradycardia symptomatic?	That depends on cardiac reserve, but frequently at rates less than 60 and almost always at rates less than 40. The ideal heart rate for maximizing cardiac output is 90.
What are some mechanisms that cause sinus bradycardia?	1. Intrinsic disease of the S-A node (SAN) and other pacemaker issues, 2° ischemia, infarction, fibrosis, and hemorrhage (e.g., sick sinus syndrome) 2. ⇑ vagal tone, 2° vomiting, micturition, pain, anxiety (commonly associated with A-V block) 3. β-blockers, Ca^{++} channel blockers, class Ia (quinidine, procainamide) and Ic (encainide, flecainide, propafenone) antiarrhythmics
What are some associated clinical syndromes?	Hypothyroidism, increased intracranial pressure, sepsis, inferior MI, hyperkalemia, hypercalcemia, after carotid surgery (stimulation of carotid sinus)

Atrioventricular (A-V) Block

Anatomic components of A-V junction?	A-V node (AVN), bundle of His, proximal portions of the bundle branches. The latter two comprise the His-Purkinje system.
ECG criteria for 1° A-V block?	PR interval greater than 0.2 msec, all P waves associated with QRS complex
Can 1° A-V block be due to infranodal disease?	Yes, although rarely. Caused by preexistent disease in two of three major fascicular branches with delayed conduction in the third; associated with a wide QRS.
Characteristics of 1° A-V block?	Most commonly due to delayed conduction through AVN, with or without delayed intra-atrial conduction due to anatomic barriers, i.e., atrial enlargement, ostium primum atrial septal defect (ASD)

ECG criteria of Mobitz type I 2° A-V block?	Intermittent dissociation between atrial and ventricular activity with variability of PR interval (reciprocal to variability of preceding RP interval) prior to nonconducted P wave
Characteristics of Mobitz type I 2° A-V block?	More likely due to A-V nodal disease, i.e., ischemia, drugs, ⇑ vagal tone; usually reversible
ECG criteria of type II 2° A-V block?	Intermittent dissociation between atrial and ventricular activity with no variability of PR or RP intervals prior to nonconducted P wave
Characteristics of Mobitz type II 2° A-V block?	More likely due to infranodal (i.e., His-Purkinje) anatomic defect in conduction. Usually fixed, irreversible defect, i.e., Ca^{++} aortic valve and/or annulus or idiopathic fibrosis of the Purkinje fibers. More likely to progress to higher degree block.
ECG criteria of 3° A-V block?	Complete A-V dissociation, i.e., variability of PR interval in association with regular RR intervals

Bundle Branch Block (BBB)

Classic ECG criteria for left (L) BBB?	Widened QRS (> 0.12 sec) with large R′ wave in V_5, V_6, I_1, and aVL
Classic ECG criteria for right (R) BBB?	Widened QRS with R′ in V_1 and wide S wave in I_1, V_1, and V_2
Differential diagnosis of QRS axis deviation?	Anterior or posterior left fascicular hemiblocks, left or right ventricular hypertrophy, inferior or high lateral MI.
How to distinguish axis deviation due to hemiblock?	1. Any QRS axis deviation associated with a Q wave is usually due to MI. 2. Left anterior fascicular hemiblock: QRS axis is less than 60° (i.e., *left* axis deviation). 3. Left posterior fascicular hemiblock: QRS axis is more positive than 120° (i.e., *right* axis deviation). 4. Also with either hemiblock, QRS complex is usually less than 0.12 msec.

Can a BBB be 2° to ischemia?	This is unusual. An AVN block can result from acute ischemia, but BBB is more likely to be associated with a completed large infarct.
Other diseases associated with BBB?	Rheumatic fever, calcific aortic stenosis, scleroderma, rheumatoid arthritis, systemic lupus erythematosus, sarcoidosis, amyloidosis, endocarditis

Pharmacologic Treatment of Bradycardia

First drug of choice?	Atropine
Mechanism of action?	Parasympatholytic$\Rightarrow \Uparrow$ AVN conduction, enhance escape pacemaker function
Dose?	One ampule is 0.5 mg in 1 ml (0.5 mg/ml). Initial dose for bradycardia is 0.5 mg; for asystole, use 1 mg IV. Repeat in 2–3 minutes if no response.
Side effects?	May use liberally. Anticholinergic effects: dry mouth, dilated pupils, blurred vision due to paralysis of accommodation, urinary retention, and constipation. Doses less than 0.4 mg can cause paradoxical worsening of bradycardia. Otherwise, a safe drug with a short half-life.
Second choice?	Isoproterenol
Mechanism of action?	Almost pure β-agonist. Has both chronotropic and inotropic effects on the myocardium.
Dose?	Given as an IV infusion 0.01–0.1 μg/kg/min or 1–10 μg/min of a 1 mg/250 ml D_5W solution. Titrate to desired heart rate.
Side effects?	Onset of action within minutes; however, may increase ventricular irritability and oxygen consumption, thereby predisposing to ventricular fibrillation

Treatment if no response to atropine or isoproterenol?	Temporary pacing (see following)

Electrical Treatment of Bradycardia

Methods?	Atrial, ventricular, or atrioventricular sequential pacing
Advantages of atrial or sequential pacing?	Maintain atrial component of ventricular filling, which can contribute to 20%–30% of cardiac output, especially in noncompliant ventricles.
Routes to obtain pacing capacity?	Atrial and/or ventricular wires placed on the epicardium at the time of cardiac surgery, transvenous ventricular pacing catheter, transcutaneous pacing patches, transthoracic placement of ventricular pacing wires (in dire emergency only!)
Prerequisites to successful atrial pacing?	A-V conduction must be intact; atrium must be captured (i.e., ineffective during atrial flutter, atrial fibrillation).
Which bradycardias respond to atrial pacing?	1. Sinus bradycardia 2. Slow junctional rhythm
Which bradycardias require A-V pacing?	1. Complete heart block 2. Second-degree heart block (to achieve 1:1 conduction) 3. First-degree heart block with markedly prolonged PR interval
Which bradycardias require ventricular pacing?	1. Afib/flutter with slow ventricular response 2. Failure of capture of atrial pacing

TACHYARRHYTHMIAS

Classification, Etiology, and Diagnosis

What are the physiologic disadvantages of tachycardia?	1. Shortened diastole, which compromises ventricular filling and subsequently stroke volume 2. Increased myocardial oxygen consumption 3. Decreased time for coronary perfusion during diastole

What are some of the causes of tachyarrhythmias?

1. Myocardial ischemia/infarction, preexistent disease
2. Respiratory problems (endotracheal tube misplacement and irritation, hypoxia, hypercarbia, acidosis, pneumothorax)
3. Electrolyte imbalance ($\Uparrow K^+$, $\Downarrow K^+$, $\Downarrow Mg^+$); intracardiac lines (i.e., Swan-Ganz catheter)
4. Drugs
5. Hypothermia
6. Stress responses to fever, pain, fear
7. Gastric dilatation

How do you assess the patient with tachycardia?

12-lead ECG (critical to have old ECG if available), blood gas, chest x-ray, chem 10, physical exam, history, i.e., anxiety or pain?

What are five questions to be answered by ECG (especially for tachycardias)?

1. Is there a normal sinus beat (especially for tachycardias)?
2. What are the atria doing?
3. What are the ventricles doing?
4. Is there A-V dissociation?
5. What are the characteristics of onset, termination, and response to interventions (usually vagal stimulation)?

Anatomic sites of origin of tachycardias?

1. Atrium
   Sinus tachycardia
   Atrial fibrillation
   Atrial flutter
   Premature atrial contractions
   Paroxysmal atrial tachycardia
2. A-V junction
   A-V node reentrant tachycardia
   A-V junctional tachycardia
3. Ventricle
   Ventricular tachycardia
   Ventricular fibrillation
   Premature ventricular contractions

Electrophysiologic mechanism?

Reentry or increased automaticity. Most clinically important tachycardias are due to reentry (afib, monomorphic vtach, vfib, A-V node reentry).

What is reentry?

In the presence of a unidirectional block in the conduction pathway, a propagating impulse does not die out but continues to reactivate the heart because the activation wavefront always encounters excitable tissue.

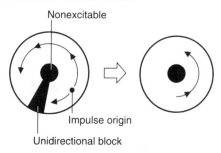

Nonexcitable

Impulse origin

Unidirectional block

What is the carotid response?

Direct, steady pressure of 5–10 seconds' duration over the carotid sinus stimulates fibers of the vagus nerve, which increases vagal tone to the heart, thereby decreasing rate of impulse formation in the SA node and other pacemaker tissues and slowing A-V nodal conduction.

Requirements for carotid massage?

Supine patient, ECG monitoring, IV access

Contraindications to carotid massage?

Carotid bruit is a relative contraindication. Never perform simultaneous bilateral carotid massage!

How can the carotid response help determine the etiology of tachycardia?

Sinus tach—slowing and reacceleration of rate

A-V node reentry—often terminates the arrhythmia.

Ventricular tachycardia—when associated with retrograde A-V node conduction, carotid massage can slow the rate of retrograde atrial activation, which manifests on ECG as a change in the rate of P waves seen after each QRS in the ST segments.

Afib/flutter—can slow ventricular response enough to better characterize atrial activity.

Do accessory pathways respond to carotid massage?

No! Hence, a slowing of the ventricular rate in response to carotid massage rules out the presence of an accessory pathway.

What are narrow complex tachycardias?

The QRS complex is less than or equal to 0.12 sec, meaning that the ventricles are activated in an orderly, swift manner through the A-V junction. These are always supraventricular in origin, i.e., atrial or A-V junctional.

What are wide complex tachycardias?

The QRS complex is greater than 0.12 sec, implying activation of the ventricles in a less orderly, slower manner. Can be supraventricular (with aberrant conduction) or ventricular in origin.

What is aberrancy?

Abnormally slow or rapid activation of the ventricles

What is a common initiating arrhythmia for vtach?

Premature ventricular contractions (PVCs)

What is a common initiating arrhythmia for A-V node reentry?

Premature atrial contractions (PACs) or PVCs

What is a common initiating arrhythmia for paroxysmal atrial tachycardia?

PACs

SPECIFIC TACHYCARDIAS AND THEIR TREATMENT

Sinus Tachycardia

What is it?

The normal response to certain stimuli. Defined as a heart rate greater than 100/min but usually less than 130. Higher, regular rates suggest supraventricular tachycardia or atrial flutter with 2:1 block.

Physiologic causes of sinus tachycardia?	Fever, pain, hypoxia, hypovolemia, low cardiac output, pulmonary embolus, anemia, adrenergic rebound after β-blocker withdrawal, hypermetabolic states (e.g., sepsis), gastric dilatation
Treatment?	Treat underlying cause plus sedation/analgesia. If none is found and tachycardia persists, may give β-blocker (esmolol infusion or propranolol).

Atrial Fibrillation/Flutter

What is a major goal of treatment?	To control ventricular response, not necessarily to restore sinus rhythm
Etiology?	Atrial distension (volume overload), adrenergic rebound in patients taking β-blockers preoperatively, hypoxia, ⇓ K^+
Who needs to be treated?	Essentially all patients with a rapid ventricular response or those with a noncompliant ventricle who need atrial systole for optimal preload
Are all treated the same?	No. It is useful to triage patients into one of three levels of urgency. Level I: pulse 120–140, BP > 100, no symptoms Level II: pulse > 40, BP 80–100, dizzy, +/− angina Level III: pulse > 140, BP < 80, angina, ⇓ mental status
Treatment?	Level I/II patients are given digoxin; level II patients need a more rapid reduction of ventricular rate with β-blockers or Ca^{++} channel blockers; level III patients require emergent cardioversion.
Why digoxin?	It is the only drug available to slow ventricular response without decreasing myocardial contractility.

Disadvantages of digoxin?	1. Increases atrial conduction velocity and excitability and can convert flutter to fibrillation or increase fibrillation rate 2. Digoxin toxicity if K^+ < 4.0
Digoxin dose?	Total loading dose of 1.0–1.25 mg is usually adequate. Initial dose is 0.5 mg IV with 0.25 mg every 6 hours for two or three more doses. Should not be given within 2 hours of previous dose. Maintain on 0.125–0.25 mg PO qd.
Do digoxin levels correlate with efficacy?	Very little in the context of acute fibrillation. Ventricular response is the best indicator of adequacy. Aim for ventricular response of less than 120.
Dosing β-blockers in setting of afib?	Metoprolol 5 mg IV q 5 min. Esmolol 0.25–0.5mg/kg IV, then 50–200 μg/kg/min (short half-life, minimizes risk of adverse effects, i.e., bronchospasm, ventricular dysfunction, excessive bradycardia)
Dosing Ca⁺⁺ blockers?	Diltiazem 0.25 mg/kg over 2 minutes, then 0.35 mg/kg 15 minutes later, followed by an infusion of 10–15 mg/h. Less hypotension associated with diltiazem than with verapamil. Verapamil 2.5–5 mg IV q 15 minutes until pulse is less than 120 (much shorter half-life than diltiazem, negative inotrope, and vasodilator)
Risks of Ca⁺⁺ blockers given concomitantly with β-blockers?	Complete heart block; therefore, avoid giving β-blockers with Ca⁺⁺ blockers!
What pharmacologic agents are used to convert to sinus rhythm?	1. Type IA agents: procainamide, quinidine. Effective in converting to sinus rhythm in 60% of patients. Patients must be digitalized before conversion due to the vagolytic effect of both drugs. 2. Magnesium sulfate: 50% success for both flutter and fibrillation 3. Type IC agents: propafenone, flecainide

Nonpharmacologic conversion to sinus rhythm?	DC cardioversion at 50–100 J for fibrillation and 10–20 J for flutter. Begin digitalization immediately afterward to prevent recurrence. Rapid atrial pacing can convert type I atrial flutter (rate less than 350). All elective electrical conversion should be done with the patient on a type IA antiarrhythmic agent.
Is systemic heparinization required for cardioversion?	Yes, if fibrillation or flutter has been present for more than 24 hours (increased risk for atrial thrombus and subsequent embolization)

Premature Atrial Contractions

What arrhythmia do PACs often precede?	Afib/flutter. Unlike PVCs, they do not predict malignant ventricular arrhythmias.
Treatment?	Usually not needed, but if concern over development of afib/flutter is great enough, prophylactic digitalization is warranted. Digoxin decreases PAC frequency and slows A-V conduction if afib does occur.
Is pacing useful for PACs?	Atrial pacing at a higher rate can suppress PACs but can also trigger atrial arrhythmias.

Paroxysmal Atrial Tachycardia and A-V Node Reentry Tachycardia (PSVT)

Typical ventricular response rate?	150–250 beats/minute.
Important etiology of PAT?	Digoxin toxicity, usually associated with unidirectional A-V block
Differential diagnosis?	Sinus tachycardia, atrial flutter with 2:1 block. An esophageal atrial electrode may help diagnosis.

Treatment?	1. DC cardioversion if hemodynamic compromise is present. 2. Rapid atrial pacing can convert to sinus rhythm. 3. Carotid massage can convert A-V node reentry. 4. Ca^{++} channel blockers can convert 90% of A-V node reentry tachycardias. 5. Adenosine, 6 mg, can terminate A-V node reentry.

A-V Junctional Rhythm and Nonparoxysmal A-V Junctional Tachycardia

Typical A-V junctional rhythm?	Occurs at rates less than 60/minute
Treatment?	1. Atrial or A-V pacing, depending on the integrity of the A-V node 2. Chronotropic drugs to stimulate sinus node rates
Typical rate of nonparoxysmal A-V junctional tachycardia?	70–130/minute. Commonly associated with digitalis toxicity
Treatment?	D/C digoxin, K^+, and digibind for severe cases of digitalis toxicity. Overdrive pacing may help.

Premature Ventricular Contractions

How are they more dangerous than PACs?	Usually associated with a decrease in cardiac output and predictive of malignant ventricular arrhythmias
Etiology?	1. Myocardial ischemia/infarction 2. Hypoxia/acidosis 3. ⇓K^+ 4. Catecholamines 5. Digitalis toxicity
Who should be treated?	Aggressive treatment is warranted in early postoperative period for coronary bypass patients if overall cardiac function is impaired.

Treatment?

1. Correct serum K$^+$ (may need > 4.5 mEq/L)
2. Atrial pace at rate greater than sinus rhythm
3. Lidocaine 1 mg/kg IV with additional boluses of 0.5 mg/kg, then drip 1–2 mg/min
4. Load procainamide 100 mg IV q 5 min to 500–1000 mg; then infuse at 2–4 mg/min.

Side effects of lidocaine?

1. Seizures at doses higher than 4 mg/min
2. Cardiac depressant

Ventricular Tachycardia/Fibrillation

Etiology?

1. Myocardial ischemia/infarction
2. Myocardial reperfusion injury (after percutaneous transluminal coronary angioplasty [PTCA], thrombolysis, coronary artery bypass graft [CABG])
3. Ventricular aneurysm

Can ventricular tachycardia be tolerated?

Occasionally, but the increased myocardial oxygen consumption associated with this arrhythmia mandates that this rhythm eventually be converted either pharmacologically or electrically. This rhythm is inherently unstable.

Can ventricular fibrillation be tolerated?

Never! Defibrillate immediately.

Treatment of sustained (more than 30 seconds) ventricular tachycardia?

Easy. If hemodynamically stable ⇒ lidocaine followed by procainamide as in PVCs. If unstable ⇒ cardioversion.

What settings for defibrillation?

Initially 200 J, then 300 J, followed by 360 J if unsuccessful

What if no response to defibrillation?

Epinephrine 1 mg IV (10 ml of a 1:10,000 solution)

Alternative treatments?

1. Ventricular overdrive pacing can break reentry circuit.
2. Bretylium 5 mg/kg bolus IV, then 10 mg/kg q 5 min, to a total dose of 30 mg, followed by a 2 mg/min drip
3. Don't use bretylium in postop patients.

What is torsades de pointes?	A form of nonsustained polymorphic ventricular tachycardia that is particularly prone to ventricular fibrillation
Risk factors for torsades?	Class IA antiarrythmics, $\Downarrow K^+$, $\Downarrow Mg^{++}$, tricyclic antidepressants
Treatment of torsades?	D/C offending drug, $\Uparrow K^+$ and Mg^{++}, ventricular or atrial pacing at 80–120 beats/minute or atropine isoproteronol to increase heart rate

The Defibrillator

What is the difference between cardioversion and defibrillation?	Both entail delivery of a depolarizing impulse. However, cardioversion is synchronized to the patient's ECG, whereas defibrillation is asynchronous.
What is the "vulnerable period?"	Corresponds to the T wave after depolarization. Delivery of an impulse during this period runs the risk of inducing ventricular fibrillation. Synchronized impulses are fired during the R wave.
What is the risk of inducing fibrillation using asynchronous cardioversion?	From 2%–5%, so you can use it in an emergency if unable to synchronize with patient's rhythm.
What rhythms should synchronous cardioversion be used for?	All arrhythmias except ventricular fibrillation. Some ventricular tachycardias are difficult to synchronize and require asynchronous cardioversion.
Is anesthesia required for cardioversion?	Yes, for elective cases but not for emergencies
Is defibrillation useful for cardiac standstill?	Absolutely not. Only if you cannot distinguish standstill from fine fibrillation is defibrillation justified.

What energy settings do you use?	Atrial fibrillation: 50–100 J (synchronous) Atrial flutter: 10 –25 J (synchronous) Ventricular tachycardia: 50–360 J (may be asynchronous if necessary) Ventricular fibrillation: 200–360 J (asynchronous)

MANAGEMENT OF CARDIAC ARREST IN THE ICU

First step?	Airway, breathing: hand ventilate with 100% oxygen at 15–20 breaths/minute, auscultate for bilateral breath sounds, intubate if necessary, and place chest tubes if necessary.
Next?	Assess cardiac rhythm.
Treatment for vfib/ pulseless vtach?	Defibrillation at 200/300/360 J
If no response after defib, what next?	Epinephrine, 1 mg IV (ml of 1:10,000 solution)
Lidocaine dose?	1–1.5 mg/kg bolus followed by 0.5–0.75 mg/kg boluses q 5 minutes until a total dose of 3 mg/kg; then infuse 2–4 mg/min.
When to use procainamide?	For ventricular ectopy or sustained Vtach if lidocaine is not successful, start with 20–30 mg/minute until rhythm is suppressed, blood pressure drops, or QRS widens 50%; then run 1–4 mg/min.
When to use bretylium?	When lidocaine and procainamide fail, use bolus with 5 mg/kg, followed by 10 mg/kg q 5 minutes to total of 30 mg/kg; then run 2 mg/minute. Don't use bretylium in postop hearts.
Treatment of asystole?	Transcutaneous pacing, epinephrine bolus 1 mg q 3–5 minutes, or atropine 1 mg IV
What is electromechanical dissociation (EMD)?	Absence of detectable blood pressure in presence of organized rhythm on the ECG

Clinical syndromes associated with EMD and their treatments?	Hypovolemia, hypoxia, cardiac tamponade, tension pneumothorax, massive A-V (PE), massive acute MI

Aortic Dissection

What is an aortic dissection?	Blood, under pressure, dissects in the level of the media separating intima and adventitia.
What is the common underlying pathophysiology of aortic dissection?	Degeneration of the aortic medial layer (medial necrosis)
What is the most common acute catastrophe of the aorta?	Acute aortic dissection. It is more common than a ruptured abdominal aortic aneurysm (AAA).
Management of suspected acute aortic dissection?	1. Insert urinary and arterial catheters. 2. Antihypertensive therapy: nitroprusside to lower mean and systolic arterial pressures, β-blocker to decrease dp/dt (e.g., esmolol or propranolol). Proceed to aortography after vital signs stable; if patient develops a complication and/or becomes unstable, proceed immediately to surgery.
Which dissections may be managed medically?	Uncomplicated descending aortic dissections; uncomplicated chronic dissections
Which should receive surgery?	All ascending dissections, all complicated dissections (e.g., those associated with rupture, visceral or limb ischemia, aortic insufficiency), inability to control pain or blood pressure medically

Coronary Blood Flow and Myocardial Oxygen Consumption

What are the three major determinants of myocardial oxygen demand?	Myocardial wall tension (30% of total), contractility, and heart rate

How is wall tension estimated clinically?	Wall tension is determined by preload, afterload, and compliance, which partly determines chamber size when the heart is filling, is estimated by left atrial pressure (LAP) or left ventricular end-diastolic pressure (LVEDP). Afterload, or the pressure in the left ventricle during contraction, is estimated by systolic blood pressure or systolic ventricular pressure.
What are the two major determinants of myocardial oxygen supply?	Arterial oxygen content and coronary blood flow
Define coronary blood flow.	Coronary blood flow = coronary perfusion pressure (CPP)/coronary vascular resistance (CVR). CVR is determined by the degree of coronary artery stenosis, as well as metabolic, hormonal, and autonomic nervous system parameters.
Most coronary blood flow occurs during which phase of the cardiac cycle?	Diastole
What is the normal resting coronary artery blood flow?	80 ml/100 g/min, or 3%–5% of cardiac output
When is myocardial wall tension highest?	During isovolumic systole
What is the most common acute catastrophe of the aorta?	Acute aortic dissection. It is more common than a ruptured AAA.

Intra-Aortic Balloon Counterpulsation

What is it?	Balloon catheter placed in descending thoracic aorta, synchronized inflation/deflation timed to cardiac rhythm
How does the IABP work?	The balloon deflates on systole, causing a fall in systemic vascular resistance (SVR), thereby decreasing the afterload on the heart. The balloon inflates on diastole, allowing for diastolic augmentation of blood pressure and

coronary perfusion. IABP is the only way to reduce afterload without reducing coronary perfusion pressure, therefore increasing myocardial oxygen delivery but decreasing myocardial oxygen demand. Conversely, inotropic agents increase cardiac output but *increase* oxygen demand as well.

How does the console driving the balloon ensure proper timing of balloon inflation and deflation?

The balloon can be timed with either the ECG or with the dicrotic notch of the central arterial waveform.

What three things does IABP do to augment cardiac performance?

1. Increases O_2 supply: inflates at peak of T wave or at dicrotic notch on A-line tracing to increase diastolic coronary and systemic perfusion by 10–15 mm Hg
2. Decreases O_2 demand: decreases afterload by deflating just prior to the R wave or pacer spike just prior to cardiac contraction
3. Increases cardiac output: increases stroke volume by as much as the size of the balloon volume used (usually 40 ml)

How does IABP reduce myocardial oxygen consumption?

By rapidly deflating just prior to systole. The aortic valve opens at 10%–15% lower pressures, thereby decreasing the maximal wall tension during isovolumic systole.

What is the diastolic pressure-time index?

The difference between aortic and left ventricular pressures during diastole (a marker of coronary perfusion). IABP insufflation during diastole increases the index (and coronary flow) by elevating aortic diastolic pressures.

Indications for IABP (in decreasing order of frequency)?

1. Postcardiotomy cardiogenic shock (35%–40%)
2. Medically refractory angina (15%–25%)
3. Preop stabilization after failed PTCA
4. Preop stabilization after acute MI
5. Complications of acute MI (mitral

regurgitation [MR], ventricular septal defect [VSD])
6. Bridge to cardiac transplantation
7. Prophylactically for induction of high-risk patients (rarely done)

Contraindications?

1. Moderate-to-severe aortic insufficiency
2. Aortic dissection. Thoracic aortic aneurysm is a relative contraindication. (Thrombolytics/anticoagulants are not contraindications.)

Can IABP be used safely in children?

Yes, smaller catheters are available and effective.

How many lumens are in a catheter?

All have one for insufflation/deflation of the balloon. Usually there is a second, central lumen as well.

What is the second lumen of a double-lumen IABP catheter used for?

For catheter placement over a guidewire (a safer technique in patients with severe vascular disease as single-lumen catheters are blindly advanced into an introducer sheath), and for proximal aortic pressure monitoring (more accurate than radial or femoral pressure tracings for synchronization).

What are the different options for IABP insertion?

1. Percutaneously into femoral artery (most common)
2. Open femoral artery cutdown
3. Suprainguinal approach to iliac artery
4. Transthoracic approach to ascending thoracic aorta
5. Open axillary artery cutdown

When is surgical placement indicated?

1. Severe iliofemoral atherosclerotic disease (option 2 > 3, > 4, > 5)
2. Aortic occlusion or severe aortoiliac disease (option 4, 5)
3. Small adults, children (option 2)
4. Heart transplant candidate who is potentially ambulatory (option 3, 5)

What two inputs are most commonly used to properly synchronize IABP?

ECG and the arterial pressure waveform

When should balloon insufflation begin?

At the peak of the T wave or just before the arterial waveform dicrotic notch

When should balloon deflation begin?

Just after the P wave (immediately before the QRS complex) or at the upswing of the arterial pulse

What are the consequences of:
   Early inflation?

Early aortic valve closure = impaired stroke volume

   Late inflation?

Poor augmentation of coronary perfusion

   Early deflation?

Poor reduction of afterload

   Late deflation?

Increased afterload = increased O_2 consumption

Identify the following:

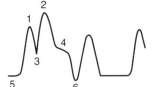

1. Unassisted peak systolic pressure
2. Augmented aortic diastolic pressure
3. Balloon inflation at dicrotic notch
4. Balloon deflation just before contraction
5. Unassisted aortic end-diastolic pressure
6. Balloon-assisted aortic end-diastolic pressure (should be lower than 5)
7. Balloon-assisted peak systolic pressure

Is the assisted aortic diastolic pressure always higher than the systolic pressure?

No, not if the left ventricular function is good (as in medically refractory angina).

Does pacing interfere with ECG synchronization?

Yes; if unipolar atrial pacing is used, the pacing spike may be interpreted as the QRS complex. Most consoles are compatible with bipolar ventricular pacing.

What is the maximum rate for 1:1 synchronization?

150/minute. For ventricular rates higher than this, use 1:2 synchronization.

What is the lowest synchronization ratio?

1:4. Any lower and you risk thrombus formation on quiescent balloon.

Complications of IABP

What are the most catastrophic (fortunately very rare) complications of IABP?

1. Aortic dissection/rupture
2. Iliofemoral dissection/rupture
3. CNS embolization (including paraplegia)

Mechanism of dissection?

Catheter tip erodes through ulcerated plaque.

Most common complication?

Distal limb ischemia (occurs to some degree in 5%–15%); 5% of these will require operative repair, usually patch angioplasty or femoral-femoral bypass.

Mechanism of ischemia?

Thrombosis or distal embolization; hence, you must frequently monitor distal pulses in any patient with an intra-aortic balloon in place.

Other complications?

Local infection, hemorrhage at the site of insertion, A-V fistula, or pseudoaneurysm formation

Differential diagnosis of diminished distal pulses in patient on IABP?

Hypothermia, ⇓ cardiac output, pressors (vasoconstriction), or acute ischemia

Treatment of acute ischemia?

1. Remove introducer sheath; or
2. Remove catheter if hemodynamically stable; or
3. Replace catheter in contralateral limb if unstable, using smaller sheath; or
4. Femoral-femoral bypass with transthoracic placement if unstable

Is visceral ischemia a problem?

Renal ischemia secondary to emboli is not uncommon. Mesenteric ischemia, however, is rare.

Diagnosis of balloon rupture?

Blood in pneumatic line, loss of diastolic pressure augmentation

Nonvascular complications?	Thrombocytopenia (secondary to balloon trauma or concomitant heparin), line infection, sepsis

Weaning IABP

Criteria for weaning?	1. Normal platelets 2. Normal coagulation parameters 3. Hemodynamically stable on minimal inotropes (< 5 μg/kg/minute dopamine)
Operative or nonoperative removal?	Surgical placement = surgical removal; otherwise pull it when ready.
Algorithm for weaning?	Stop heparin for 4–6 hours, change synchronization ratio to 1:2, wait 4 hours; if stable, decrease ratio to 1:4; remove if stable. Allow brief (3–4 beats) flash of blood to flush out debris; then keep firm pressure over arteriotomy site for 30–45 minutes.
Is decreasing the synchronization ratio the only way to wean?	No. Alternatively you can decrease the volume of the balloon from 40→ 30 → 20 ml.
Where do you position the IABP?	Approximately 3 cm distal to the left subclavian takeoff and above renal arteries. You need a chest x-ray to confirm. Adjust as needed. Tip should be about at the level of the carina.
If patient goes into afib or requires pacing, does IABP need to be turned off and/or removed?	No, the IABP can trigger either from the ECG or the patient's arterial waveform; triggering from A-line waveform optimizes performance in these settings.
Where should you compress an artery after removing an IABP (or any other arterial catheter)?	At 1–2 cm proximal to the skin puncture site. (Remember, the needle enters the skin at an angle, i.e., the arterial puncture site is proximal to the skin site.)

HEART FAILURE

What is the common feature explaining dyspnea in all types (dilated, hypertrophic, restrictive) of cardiomyopathies?	Elevated left atrial pressure → increased pulmonary venous pressure with resultant edema and decreased oxygenation

List some potentially reversible causes of a "dilated" cardiomyopathy.

1. Alcoholic cardiomyopathy
2. Hypocalcemia, hypokalemia, hypophosphatemia
3. Hemochromatosis
4. Pheochromocytoma
5. Myocarditis
6. Sarcoid heart disease
7. Lead poisoning
8. Selenium deficiency
9. Uremic cardiomyopathy
10. Ischemic cardiomyopathy
11. Pregnancy

Name six ways to alter cardiac output. (Remember CO = HR × SV.)

1. Heart rate (pacing, inotropes)
2. Preload (fluids, decrease intrathoracic pressure)
3. Afterload (vasodilators, IABP)
4. Contractility (inotropes)
5. Compliance (making heart nonischemic, relief of tamponade)
6. Rate and rhythm (i.e., treat afib to regain 25%–30% of cardiac output; make rhythm regular for optimal performance; optimal rate is about 90)

What are the classic physical signs of ventricular dysfunction?

1. Distended neck veins
2. Lateral point of maximal impulse (PMI)
3. S_3 gallop
4. Murmurs of mitral regurgitation and/or tricuspid regurgitation
5. Rales
6. Distended ± pulsatile liver
7. Edema (peripheral and sacral).
These signs are helpful only when positive; i.e., patients may have significant heart failure without a gallop, rales, etc.

What is the significance of narrow pulse pressures in patients with cardiomyopathies?	Associated with a CI less than 2 l/min/m^2
What are common inotropic agents?	• β-agonists (dobutamine, epinephrine, dopamine, isoproterenol) • Phosphodiesterase inhibitors (milrinone, amrinone) • Digoxin
Can different inotropic agents be used together?	Yes. β-agonists, phosphodiesterase inhibitors, and digoxin all work through different pathways and can thus have additive effects.
What are potential cardiovascular side effects of inotropic medications?	1. Arrhythmias (e.g., sinus tachycardia, ventricular tachycardia, ventricular fibrillation) 2. Hypotension (Many agents cause vasodilation.) 3. Tolerance (The drugs can become ineffective, a process called tachyphylaxis.)
What are angiotensin converting enzyme (ACE) inhibitors used for?	First-line therapy for any patient with a reduced ejection fraction
What are some potential side effects of ACE inhibitors?	1. Hypotension 2. Renal failure (patients with bilateral renal artery stenosis) 3. Hyperkalemia 4. Allergic reactions (the most serious is angioedema) 5. Cough
If ACE inhibitors are not tolerated, what drug combination is generally used?	Hydralazine and isosorbide
What are the three basic physiologic causes of hypotension?	A drop in preload, afterload, or contractility
What drugs can be used to improve contractility?	Dopamine, dobutamine, epinephrine, norepinephrine, and milrinone

What drugs can be used to augment afterload?	Phenylephrine, dopamine, norepinephrine, epinephrine
What can be done to augment preload?	Volume expansion
How is the mechanism of action of milrinone different from that of the other agents used to improve contractility?	Milrinone acts as a phosphodiesterase inhibitor, causing the intracellular accumulation of cyclic adenosine monophosphate (cAMP). The other agents work through activating the β receptor. Therefore, in the failing myocardium, a combination of both agents may be beneficial.
What is the difference between nitroglycerin and nitroprusside?	Nitroglycerin is primarily a dilator of capacitance vessels, whereas nitroprusside acts primarily on resistance vessels.

Acute MI

What is the most common cause of mortality postoperatively in patients undergoing carotid endarterectomy?	MI
Name three cardiac isoenzymes.	1. CK [creatine kinase, myocardial band (MB) fraction] 2. LDH (lactate dehydrogenase) 3. AST (asparate aminotransferase)
Name seven causes of CK elevation.	1. Acute MI 2. Myocarditis 3. Trauma/status epilepticus/surgery 4. Severe, prolonged exercise 5. Polymyositis/muscular dystrophy 6. Devastating brain injury 7. Familial elevation
Name three causes of CK-MB elevation.	1. Acute MI 2. Cardiac surgery 3. Muscular dystrophy
Name four causes of CK-BB elevation (brain fraction).	1. Brain injury/Reye's syndrome 2. Uremia 3. Malignant hyperthermia 4. Small intestinal necrosis

Name several causes of LDH elevation.	1. Acute MI 2. Pernicious anemia/sickle cell crisis 3. Large PE 4. Renal infarction 5. Prosthetic heart valves 6. Hemolytic anemia 7. Liver injury
Which isoenzyme elevates first following an acute MI?	• CK/CKMB (within 6 hours depending on the assay) • LDH is elevated within 24 hours.
What is the prognostic significance of ventricular fibrillation early after an acute MI (hours to days)?	None
What is the prognostic significance of ventricular fibrillation late after an acute MI (days)?	Significant increase in mortality; this requires evaluation and treatment. This event suggests persistent ischemia.
What are the common thrombolytic agents?	1. Tissue plasminogen activator (tPA) 2. Streptokinase (SK) 3. Anosylated plasminogen streptokinase activator complex (APSAC) 4. Urokinase (UK)
What are some contraindications to thrombolysis?	1. Recent trauma/surgery (active bleeding) 2. Recent stroke 3. Significant hypertension 4. Recent history of chest compressions
What are other important medications used in the treatment of an MI?	1. Aspirin 2. β blockers 3. Nitrates 4. Narcotics
List two causes of a new murmur after an acute MI.	1. MR 2. VSD
How can you make this differentiation?	1. Auscultation; frequently not helpful as both are holosystolic murmurs; however, a VSD is usually heard best over the sternum. The MR murmur can be heard at the apex but frequently radiates superiorly in

posterior leaflet/papillary muscle ruptures, and posteriorly in anterior leaflet/papillary muscle ruptures.
2. ECG/Doppler
3. Right heart catheterization with measurement of the oxygen saturation in the various chambers. An increase in oxygen saturation by more than 5% between chambers is consistent with a shunt.

    e.g., RAO_2 saturation 61%
    RVO_2 saturation 75%
    PAO_2 saturation 78%
    Arterial saturation 95%
    Consistent with a VSD

Can the amount of L → R shunting be *estimated* in a VSD (or ASD)?

Yes. Variables needed include arterial O_2 saturation (ART sat), RAO_2 saturation (RA sat), and PAO_2 saturation (sat).

Shunt (Qp/Qs) = (ART sat – RA sat) ÷ (ART sat – PA sat)

From above, Qp/Qs = (95 – 61) ÷ (95 – 78) = 2/1 shunt; i.e., there is twice as much pulmonary blood flow compared with systemic blood flow with the shunt at the RV level.

List six mechanical complications after an acute MI.

1. Left ventricular aneurysm
2. Left ventricular rupture
    free wall contained = pseudoaneurysm
    noncontained = death
    septal = VSD
3. Papillary muscle rupture (acute mitral regurgitation)
4. Thromboembolus
5. Reinfarction/extension
6. Pericardial effusion/tamponade

List five causes of chest pain after an acute MI.

1. Reinfarction
2. Infarct extension
3. Recurrent ischemia
4. Pericarditis
5. Noncardiac (e.g., GI)

What is the first therapy for hypotension/shock associated with an acute MI?

• Vasopressors/inotropes
• Hemodynamic monitoring

Electrocardiogram

Name some causes of ST elevation.

1. Acute MI
2. Ventricular aneurysm
3. Pericarditis
4. Myocardial contusion
5. Prinzmetal's angina
6. Early repolarization
7. Hypothermia (Osbourne J wave)
8. Hyperkalemia
9. Artifact

(Occasionally seen with LBBB, left ventricular hypertrophy, myocardial neoplasms, hypertrophic myopathies)

Name five causes of ST depression.

1. Acute *posterior* MI
2. Ischemia
3. Digoxin
4. Left ventricular hypertrophy
5. BBBs

Name some important causes of T-wave inversion.

1. Ischemia
2. Electrolyte abnormalities
3. Medications (digoxin)
4. BBBs
5. Myocarditis
6. With subarachnoid hemorrhages
7. After a ventricular premature beat (VPB) and some tachycardias

Name some causes of ectopy (atrial and ventricular).

1. Ischemia
2. Reperfusion after thrombolytic therapy (the classic example is AIVR—accelerated idioventricular rhythm, also known as slow VT)
3. Electrolytes (K^+, MG^{++}, Ca^{++}) abnormalities
4. Hypoxia
5. Monitoring lines (e.g., Swan-Ganz catheters, CVP lines)
6. Medications (β agonists, antiarrhythmics)
7. Endogenous catechols (pain, anxiety)

Management of the Cardiac Transplant Patient

What medication should *not* be used to treat bradycardia after heart transplantation?	Atropine
What medications should be used to treat bradycardia after heart transplantation?	Epinephrine, isoproterenol
What medication should *not* be used to treat supraventricular tachycardias after heart transplantation?	Digoxin. The long-term use of β blockers is also generally discouraged as these agents reduce exercise tolerance.
Why are tachy-, brady-, and dysrhythmias treated differently in heart transplant recipients?	The heart is denervated; therefore, vagolytic (atropine) and vagotonic (digoxin) agents are not effective (as stated previously).
Can a heart transplant patient have a heart attack?	Yes. Coronary artery disease (CAD) is a manifestation of chronic rejection. About 50% of heart transplant patients have some evidence of CAD at 5 years; this is usually significant in only 5%.
Does reinnervation ever occur?	Yes; 75% of heart recipients show some sympathetic reinnervation after 1 year.
Does reinnervation have any practical implication?	Yes. Patients who reinnervate have improved exercise performance (faster heart rate response). Also, some recipients who develop CAD complain of chest pain (angina).
How long can a heart be stored before transplantation?	Approximately 4 hours in cold preservation solution
When are infections most common after any transplant?	The first 3–6 months

| What type of infections are most common after transplantation (other than a "cold")? | Bacterial (common), atypical bacterial, followed by viral, fungal, and protozoal |

| What organ systems are most frequently involved with cytomegalovirus (CMV)? | • GI (stomach, colon)
• Lung (pneumonitis)
• Other (heart, etc.)
CMV infections can also stimulate the immune system and, therefore, are frequently associated with rejection. |

| When is rejection most common (any organ)? | The first 1–2 months |

| What factors are important for successful heart, lung, and heart–lung transplantation? | ABO compatibility and approximate size match, short ischemic time |

| In a heart–lung transplant recipient, is it possible to reject a lung without concomitant heart rejection? | Yes. Either lung may show evidence of rejection without involvement of the opposite lung or the heart. |

Management of Postcardiac Surgical Patients

| How do you control postoperative bleeding after cardiopulmonary bypass? | Use the mnemonic 10 Ps.
Poikilothermy. Patient is cold-blooded for awhile. Cold blood won't clot. Get temperature to 37°C.
Pressure. Lower arterial pressure to 90–100 systolic. Raise head of bed to control CVP.
PEEP (7.5–10 cm H_2O). This is controversial but may put additional pressure on mammary bed in patients who have had internal mammary artery takedowns.
DDAVP (0.3 μg/kg; especially helpful in uremia)
Protamine 25 extra mg (Unreversed heparin washes out of previously underperfused vascular beds.)
Amino CaProic Acid:
Low dose = 5 g
Medium dose = 10 g
High dose = 30 g |

Use judiciously in low cardiac output state and in patient with small, diseased vessels (risk of graft thrombosis).

Platelets. The most common coagulation abnormality after cardiac surgery is platelet dysfunction.

Plasma, fresh frozen. Not very helpful except in Coumadin users.

CryoPrecipitate. Useful for factor 8 or fibrinogen deficiency.

Prolene. Sometimes the bleeding is "surgical," requiring reexploration.

How can you warm hypothermic patients?

Warm all fluids. Turn heater in vent humidifier to 40°C. Warm the room until it is like a sauna. Heat lamps shining on torso (no blankets). Decrease loss due to convection by covering bed rails with blankets (bear hugger).

How can a patient with actively draining mediastinal chest tubes after bypass develop tamponade?

Blood can collect in loculations, compressing specific parts of the heart.

How much chest tube output after cardiopulmonary bypass is too much?

It varies for each surgeon. In general, output should not be greater than 250 ml/hr × 4 hours; after 4 hours, you want less than 100 ml/hr. Once the output is less than 100 ml/hr, the bleeding will almost always stop.

Which pump cases are at greater risk for factor deficiencies/platelet dysfunction?

The ones that last more than 3 hours

Why might transthoracic pacing wires not work well after 7–10 days?

Scar and edema can cause an insulating block to prevent conduction to the myocardium.

Your patient has a Swan-Ganz PA catheter. You want to check the pulmonary capillary wedge pressure; but when you inflate the balloon, the pressure tracing rapidly increases until it is off the scale. What is happening?

The PA catheter is "overwedging." The balloon is too far into the pulmonary artery. When you inflate the balloon, it squeezes longitudinally until it covers over the pressure monitoring hole at the catheter tip. This causes the monitor trace to rise off the scale. This is a dangerous position for the PA catheter, because it greatly increases the likelihood of rupture of the PA by the balloon. To avoid this catastrophe, always inflate the balloon slowly while watching the monitor trace. If it begins to overwedge, STOP, deflate the balloon, and pull back the PA catheter before trying again.

Suppose someone hasn't read this book, overwedges the PA catheter, and ruptures the PA?

The first thing you will notice will be hemoptysis. The balloon should be carefully reinflated after pulling the catheter back a bit in an attempt to tamponade the bleeding site. The patient should be positioned with the injured side down if he is not intubated and immediately intubated, preferably with a double-lumen endotracheal tube to prevent aspiration of blood into the noninvolved side. Lacking a double-lumen tube, selective intubation of the opposite main-stem bronchus serves the same function. Stop all anticoagulation and make sure blood is available for transfusion. In severe cases, emergency surgery will be necessary.

What should you do first when a "fresh" CABG patient arrives in the ICU?

Feel the femoral pulse and visually ensure that the chest is moving with ventilation.

What questions should be asked about such a patient?

What procedure was done; any reactions to protamine or drips; rate; last hemoglobin; any problems in the OR?

What studies must be checked ASAP in the new postoperative patient?

Cardiac indices, ECG, chest x-ray, chest tube drainage, urine output

What should you check on the chest x-ray?

1. Endotracheal tube placement; it should be at about the level of clavicles.
2. Air or fluid in the pleural space
3. Pulmonary artery catheter position; this should be within mediastinal shadow.

Indications for mediastinal reexploration?

Tamponade physiology (tachycardia, high filling pressures), hypotension, decreased urine output, large chest output that stops suddenly, massive mediastinal hemorrhage (e.g., 1000 ml in 5 min), refractory asystole/vtach without a pulse. No postoperative cardiac patient should be coded without opening the chest!

Role of dopamine in most CABG patients?

Most patients come into the unit on 5 μg/kg/min of dopamine, then are rapidly weaned to renal dose (3 μg/kg/min) and stopped the morning of postoperative day 1.

What is the most common inotrope used for low CI and high SVRI after cardiac surgery?

Dobutamine

Is hetastarch an anticoagulant?

Yes. Hetastarch should be avoided in the early care of postoperative patients.

What is the order of removal of temporary pacing wires and chest tubes?

Wires first (if no arrhythmias), followed 1 hour later by chest tubes if less than 20 ml/hr of mediastinal chest tube drainage

What is the order of removal of IABP, endotracheal tube, chest tubes, wires?

1. IABP
2. Extubate
3. Wires
4. Chest tubes
5. Pulmonary artery catheter

Rx of postcardiac surgical atrial fibrillation?

One third of patients will go into atrial fibrillation after cardiopulmonary bypass. Digitalis load and then metoprolol 5 mg IV repeated until rate is controlled. Think about diuresing with furosemide to reduce atrial stretch.

Most common cause of hyponatremia in postoperative cardiopulmonary bypass patients?	Fluid overload. Use diuretics; they promote free water clearance.
What is the purpose of hemodynamic monitoring in the postoperative cardiac patient?	To assess volume status and cardiac output
What is cardiac output?	(Heart rate) × (stroke volume)
What is CI?	(Cardiac output) ÷ (body surface area)
For a postoperative cardiac patient, what CI indicates a severe reduction in cardiac output?	Less than 2.0 L/min/m^2
What is the ultimate indicator of volume status?	LVEDP
What is the best means to estimate LVEDP in an ICU patient?	Via a Swan-Ganz catheter that measures left-sided pressures by right heart catheterization
What is pulmonary capillary wedge pressure (PCWP)?	When the balloon catheter tip of the Swan-Ganz catheter wedges at a branched pulmonary artery, it measures the transmitted left atrial pressure, which most closely approximates LVEDP.
If the Swan-Ganz catheter does not wedge, what can be used to approximate LVEDP?	Pulmonary artery diastolic pressure (PAD)
When does PAD not correlate with the wedge pressure?	In severe lung disease with pulmonary vascular changes (pulmonary hypertension)
What is the most common complication seen during placement of Swan-Ganz catheters?	Arrhythmias

What is the most dreaded complication of Swan-Ganz catheters?	Pulmonary artery perforation from overwedging
What is the characteristic Swan-Ganz tracing in acute MR?	A "v" wave in the wedge tracing representing regurgitant flow into the left atrium
What is the characteristic finding in acute ventricular septal rupture?	An oxygen saturation step-up in the pulmonary artery as compared to the right atrium
What Swan-Ganz tracings are suggestive of a hemodynamically significant pulmonary embolus?	Elevated right heart pressures (CVP, PAS, PAD), with a normal wedge pressure
What does one see in cardiac tamponade?	Equilibrium of all pressures (CVP, PAD, PCWP) at a high value
A resident is performing a bedside procedure under local anesthesia. A short time after the initial subcutaneous lidocaine injection, the patient reports slight nausea and faints. The pulse rate is noted to be 26. The resident orders an immediate intravenous injection. Within 15 seconds, the patient recovers and pulse rate is 90. What drug could have corrected this problem?	Atropine 0.5–1.0 mg IV
What is the name given to the response to a simple needle stick as described in the previously mentioned patient?	Vaso-vagal reflex
What action of atropine is responsible for its correcting the problem?	It blocks vagal impulses that slow the heart rate.

What is the mixed venous oxygen saturation?

The mixed venous oxygen saturation, or SVO_2, measures the amount of oxygen left over in the blood returning to the heart. The SVO_2 reflects both oxygen delivery and oxygen extraction. Generally speaking, an SVO_2 of less than 65% is abnormal and warrants investigation.

What causes a low SVO_2 in postoperative cardiac patients?

Low cardiac output, poor arterial oxygenation, and anemia are common causes of decreased oxygen delivery. Fever and agitation are common causes of increased oxygen demand.

Your patient has been experiencing excessive chest tube drainage over the past several hours due to a coagulopathy. The drainage suddenly ceases. What should you do?

Obtain a chest x-ray. The concern is that the chest tubes have clotted, and the blood is now accumulating in the chest, a situation that can lead to cardiac tamponade. Look for a widened mediastinum or a pleural accumulation on the chest film. The chest x-ray is not a good way to make the diagnosis of tamponade, but it can provide clues as to whether blood is accumulating.

What are some causes of excess bleeding after heart surgery?

1. Technical problems, such as bleeding, from a suture line or a side branch of a vein or mammary graft
2. Excess of heparin. Diagnosis— measure prothrombin time (PTT) or the activated clotting time (ACT). Treatment—give protamine. This is a common problem when underperfused vascular beds open up postoperatively
3. Hypothermia. Cold blood won't clot. Rewarm your patient. This is a big deal.
4. Platelet dysfunction, caused by platelet contact with the cardiopulmonary bypass machine or postoperative aspirin. Diagnosis— bleeding time, platelet count. Treatment—administer DDAVP or transfuse platelets, or both.
5. Clotting factor deficiency, caused by excessive transfusion with packed RBCs or retransfusion of large

volumes of washed blood.
Diagnosis—prolonged PT.
Treatment—administer fresh frozen
plasma.

6. Fibrinolysis, caused by many factors,
   including excessive bleeding, blood
   contact with the bypass machine,
   retransfusion of shed blood.
   Diagnosis—thromboelastogram,
   decreased fibrinogen level, fibrin split
   products, or D-dimer. Treatment—
   aminocaproic acid (Amicar).

What are some clinical indicators of adequate perfusion in an ICU patient?

1. Urine output is probably the best
   clinical indicator of perfusion. A well-
   perfused adult patient should
   generally have 1 ml/kg/hr of urine
   output.
2. Feel the patient's feet and hands. A
   well-perfused patient will have warm
   extremities, with brisk (less than 1
   second) capillary refill.
3. Normal mentation is often listed as a
   sign of adequate perfusion, but many
   patients in the ICU have been given
   sedation, making this assessment
   difficult.
4. Patients with inadequate perfusion
   are often tachycardic.

What assumptions are made when equating PCWP to cardiac preload?

To know the preload, you need to know
the LVEDP. In the ICU, it is not
practical to insert a measurement
catheter into the left ventricle. The
chain of assumptions goes like this:
LVEDP ≅ PCWP. It is important to
understand when these assumptions are
not valid. The LVEDP is not necessarily
reflected by the LA pressure in the
setting of mitral stenosis, or in patients
with a stiff, noncompliant ventricle, as in
left ventricular hypertrophy. The PCWP
may not reflect the LAP in patients with
pulmonary vascular hypertension or in
patients on high PEEP.

What is the normal value for the PCWP?

12–15 mm Hg in resting adult patients
at sea level

Is the PCWP representative of the LVEDP during the first few hours after a CABG?

There may be a poor correlation between PCWP and LVEDP during this period due to a change in compliance of the left ventricle. The ventricle may be stiffer.

11 — Renal System, Fluids, and Electrolytes

What are maintenance fluid requirements?

These are based on body weight:
For the first 10 kg—100 ml/kg/day (or approximately 4 ml/kg/hr)
For the next 10 kg—50 ml/kg/day (or approximately 2 ml/kg/hr)
For weight above 20 kg—20 ml/kg/day (or approximately 1 ml/kg/hr)
Remember, infants need 4 ml/kg/hr of fluid in and at least 2 ml/kg/hr of urine out. Bigger children need 2 ml/kg/hr in and 1 ml/kg/hr out.

What can increase fluid requirements?

Remember the mnemonic **A, B, C, D, E, F**:
Air: intubated patients or those with tracheostomies who breathe unhumidified air
Burn: fluid loss through a burn or open wound can be several times the maintenance
Cavities: places to hide water that make it less available to the vascular space such as the bowel with obstruction of retroperitoneum with pancreatitis
Diarrhea
Enterocutaneous fistulas
Fever: 10% increase for each degree F increase in body temperature

How much Na⁺, K⁺, and Cl⁻ are required each day?

About 1 mEq/kg/day each

How much Ca⁺⁺ and Mg⁺⁺ are required each day in a 70-kg adult?

Ca^{++} = 2 g/day; Mg^{++} = 20 mEq/day. Neither is necessary, however, in maintenance IV fluid.

What is the standard maintenance fluid?

Dextrose (D) 5 $\frac{1}{2}$ or $\frac{1}{4}$ normal saline with 20 or 30 mEq of KCl added will provide more than enough salt and just enough potassium.

What is the normal osmolality of blood?	About 300 mOsm
What is the main endocrine regulator of osmolality and how does it work?	Antidiuretic hormone (ADH). As osmolality exceeds 300 mOsm, osmoreceptor cells in the supraoptic nuclei of the hypothalamus send the signal to the posterior hypothalamus to increase production of ADH. This increases water reabsorption from the distal renal tubules.
Why is D5 (5% dextrose) included in most maintenance fluids?	It helps to make the fluid more isotonic, and it has been shown that 100 g of glucose per day will provide enough metabolic substrate to cut protein losses in half in fasting patients.
What are the clinical findings of hypovolemia?	Thirst, decreased skin turgor, weight loss, oliguria, tachycardia, orthostatic hypotension, BUN/creatinine ratio > 20:1, increased hematocrit, urine sodium < 20 mEq/L
What is the first-line fluid therapy for hypovolemia?	Isotonic crystalloid solutions: 1. Lactated Ringer's (for resuscitation) 2. Normal saline (used more for acute replacement of known losses, but watch the sodium and chloride load)
How much of administered isotonic intravenous fluid can be expected to stay in the vascular space?	Only about $\frac{1}{3}$; the rest goes extravascular.
Are other fluids ever used in fluid resuscitation and why?	Yes. Colloid-containing solutions such as 5% and 25% albumin, Dextran, or Hetastarch are used to minimize extravascular loss and volume overload in special circumstances such as heart failure, renal failure, or pulmonary edema.
Which electrolyte is involved in the three main endocrine-mediated mechanisms of intravascular volume maintenance?	Na^+, because water follows Na^+.

What are the three main endocrine mediators of intravascular volume and how do they work?

1. Renin–angiotensin system
2. Aldosterone
3. Atrial natriuretic peptide (ANP). Decreased renal perfusion causes juxtaglomerular apparatus cells in the kidney to release renin. Renin converts plasma angiotensinogen (made by the liver) to angiotensin I, which is converted to angiotensin II by angiotensin-converting enzyme (ACE) in the lungs. Angiotensin II has a number of effects, including the increased reabsorption of Na^+, and thus water, in the renal tubules. It also stimulates the secretion of aldosterone from the adrenal cortex, which increases the number of $Na^+/K^+/ATPases$ in the tubular cells, resulting in the increased reabsorption of Na^+, and thus water, at the expense of K^+, H^+, and ATP. ANP is released from the right atrium with increased pressure and stretching. It inhibits renal reabsorption of Na^+, and thus water.

What is the most common cause of hyponatremia?

Excess free water administration. This can be from exogenous sources (hypotonic fluids) or endogenous sources (ADH). Any stress such as surgery can result in a transient form of the syndrome of inappropriate antidiuretic hormone release (SIADH), but it is classically seen with tumors and head injury.

What are the symptoms of hyponatremia?

Weakness, fatigue, headache, confusion, seizure, muscle cramps, coma

What is hyperosmolar hyponatremia?

Excess solute in the plasma space (pseudohyponatremia) such as lipid, mannitol, glucose, protein, or radiologic contrast causes the osmotic shift of water into the vascular space, causing measured Na^+ to be low.

What is the treatment of hyponatremia?

First, determine the cause. If it is mild SIADH, then restrict free water. If there is true Na⁺ depletion from GI or renal losses and/or the patient is symptomatic, then hypertonic saline should be administered to correct the Na⁺ deficit. Remember also that loop diuretics cause the excretion of free water in excess of Na⁺, thus raising the serum Na⁺.

What is the risk of correcting a sodium deficit too fast?

Central pontine myelinolysis

What is an acceptable rate of correction?

0.5 mEq/L/hr.

How does one correct a Na⁺ deficit safely?

The amount of Na⁺ required to increase the serum Na⁺ to a desired level can be calculated: Na needed (in mEq) = (target Na⁺ − actual Na⁺) × 0.6 (wt. in kg). The amount of Na needed to be infused over a certain time frame to raise the Na 0.5 mEq/hr can thus be calculated.

What are the clinical manifestations of hypernatremia?

CNS irritability: restlessness, ataxia, spasms, seizures

What are the main causes of hypernatremia?

1. Excess Na⁺ administration, such as using normal saline for maintenance fluids and Na⁺ bicarbonate in cardiac arrest situations
2. Excess free water loss (see previous discussion); also diabetes insipidus after head injury with lack of ADH secretion

What is the risk of lowering the serum Na⁺ too fast and what is an acceptable rate?

Free water should be administered at a rate such that the serum Na⁺ falls at 0.5 mEq/L/hr. If the serum Na⁺ falls faster, cerebral edema and herniation may occur.

What are the clinical manifestations of hyperkalemia?

1. Muscle—weakness
2. Heart—peaked T waves, widened QRS, prolonged PR interval, ventricular fibrillation, asystole

What are the two main causes of hyperkalemia?

1. Renal failure and, therefore, the inability to excrete dietary and exogenously administered K^+
2. Cellular release (crush injuries, reperfusion of ischemic tissue, tumor lysis, succinylcholine administration)

What is the treatment of hyperkalemia?

1. Protect the heart: $CaCl$ 1 g to stabilize membranes
2. Transiently lower serum K^+: 50 g glucose (1 amp) and 10–20 U insulin intravenously will push K^+ into cells and buy time.
3. Definitively lower serum K^+: Kayexalate PO or as enema will exchange Na^+ for K^+ and bind it to be eliminated. Dialysis can also be used to lower K^+ quickly and reliably.
4. Intravenous $NaHCO_3$: raising pH drives potassium into cells.

What are the clinical manifestations of hypokalemia?

Muscle weakness, predisposition to digitalis toxicity, cardiac arrhythmias, decreased intestinal motility

As blood pH increases, what happens to serum K^+?

It decreases as intracellular H^+ is exchanged for K^+.

Since about half of serum calcium is protein-bound, how can measured total serum calcium be corrected for hypoalbuminemia?

For every 1 g/dl that albumin is decreased, add 0.8 mg/dl to the measured serum Ca^{2+}.

What are the clinical manifestations of hypercalcemia?

1. Neurologic: personality disorders, confusion, coma
2. Muscular: fatigue, weakness
3. GI: nausea, vomiting, abdominal pain
4. Renal: stones (Remember: "Stones, bones, abdominal groans, and mental overtones.")

What is the treatment for hypercalcemia?

Saline diuresis (normal saline at 2–3 times maintenance with IV furosemide)

What are the major causes of hypercalcemia?

Hyperparathyroidism, bony metastases, tumors secreting PTH-like substances

What is the most common cause of severe hypocalcemia among surgical patients?	Hypoparathyroidism (usually transient) after thyroid or parathyroid surgery
What are the clinical manifestations of hypocalcemia?	Perioral tingling, paresthesias, muscle cramps, decreased deep tendon reflexes; Chvostek's sign—tapping the facial nerve produces contraction of the facial muscles; Trousseau's sign—induction of carpal spasm by inflating a BP cuff around the upper arm for 3 minutes.
What are the two physiologic mechanisms for regulating acid–base status?	1. Respiratory: can respond in minutes with increased ventilation to eliminate excess acid (as CO_2) 2. Renal: can eliminate excess acid or hold on to bicarbonate but requires hours to respond
What are some pharmacologic ways to manipulate acid–base status?	1. IV $NaHCO_3$ or other buffers 2. IV HCl or other acidic compounds
What is the mechanism of diabetic ketoacidosis?	Insulin deficiency results in increased free fatty acid release from adipose tissue, increased conversion of acetyl-CoA to ketoacids, and impaired metabolism of ketoacids.
What is the most common cause of lactic acidosis in the surgical ICU?	Tissue hypoxia and anaerobic metabolism due to inadequate delivery of oxygen to peripheral tissues (e.g., from heart failure, sepsis, hemorrhagic shock)
What are the three factors that can be altered to increase the delivery of oxygen to tissue, thus decreasing the anaerobic generation of lactic acid?	1. Cardiac output 2. Hematocrit 3. Arterial oxygen saturation
What is renal tubular acidosis?	Altered reabsorption of filtered bicarbonate resulting in excessive bicarbonate loss

At what point in metabolic acidosis should sodium bicarbonate be given?

Sodium bicarbonate should be given to keep pH above 7.2, since below this level, cardiovascular collapse could occur. However, it should not be routinely administered for metabolic acidosis. An overshoot phenomenon may result, with the development of metabolic alkalosis as precursor organic anions are converted to bicarbonate.

How is the anion gap calculated?

Anion gap = (serum Na^+) – (HCO^{+3} + Cl^-).

What are some causes of metabolic acidosis with an increased anion gap?

Use the mnemonic **MUDPILES:**
Methanol intoxication
Uremia
Diabetic ketoacidosis
Paraldehyde intoxication
Infection
Lactic acidosis
Ethylene glycol, **E**thanol intoxication
Salicylate intoxication

What is the distribution of total body water (TBW) in an adult?

TBW = 60% of total body weight: extracellular = 20% of total body weight (15% interstitial + 5% plasma); intracellular = 40% of total body weight.

It is time to remove the Foley catheter. The Foley balloon will not deflate due to a defective catheter. What substance instilled into the balloon will result in disruption of the latex balloon with evacuation of water in it?

Mineral oil, since this substance will destroy the integrity of the latex

What safe invasive procedure might be used to more quickly deflate the balloon of a defective Foley catheter?

Ultrasound guided fine-needle puncture of the Foley balloon

When a patient has a low urine output, what three main areas should be considered as causes?

1. Mechanical (Think of postrenal obstruction such as a problem with the catheter.)
2. Physiological. (Think in terms of the

patient's fluid status and cardiac status.)
3. Pharmacologic (Consider whether the patient has been diuretic-dependent or needs diuretics at this time.)

What are some potential causes of declining renal function in an ICU patient?

1. Contrast nephropathy
2. Systemic sepsis
3. Hypotension (either immediate or in the period just prior to the decreased urine output)
4. Medications (such as aminoglycosides)
5. Cholesterol embolization resulting from intra-aortic balloon pump placement or catheterization)

There are many formulas for helping determine whether low urine output is from a renal cause or some other cause such as low volume status or low cardiac output (called prerenal conditions). Which are the two easiest formulas to use?

1. Urine sodium. (If the urine sodium is under 20 mEq/L, the tubules are probably working reasonably well and the cause of the low urine output must be outside the kidney. Diuretics will confuse this issue since they cause a saluresis.)
2. Urine osmolality. (If the urine osmolality is more than 500, about twice that of serum osmolality, then the kidneys are concentrating the urine and they believe they are seeing volume contraction, either from hypovolemia or poor cardiac output. If the urine osmolality is around that of the serum [250–350], the tubules are not concentrating the urine and thus renal dysfunction may be occurring.)
°There are many other tests, such as the fractional excretion of sodium and the renal failure index, that are formulas and can be looked up when necessary.

What should be done if a Foley catheter cannot be placed in a patient who must be resuscitated?

A suprapubic catheter can be placed using a Seldinger technique similar to cannulation of a central vein. The bladder is just posterior and inferior to the pubic ramus. Such a catheter can be placed percutaneously and removed without incident when it is no longer needed.

What issues should be followed to maintain the health of the patient's kidneys?

1. Maintain adequate volume.
2. Maintain adequate cardiac output.
3. Watch urine output and make sure that it is close to 1 ml/kg/hr.
4. Protect the kidneys from dye loads.
5. Be careful with the use of diuretics.
6. Monitor laboratory indices of urinary function (creatinine and BUN).
7. Monitor nephrotoxic drugs (aminoglycosides, vancomycin, nonsteroidal anti-inflammatory agents).
8. Have a low threshold for using renal dose dopamine (3 μg/kg/hr).
9. Be very careful with drug dosages and renal insufficiency.
10. Never keep Foleys in place longer than they need to be.
11. Consider alkalinization of the urine if toxins such as myoglobin are suspected.

Are there any mechanical causes of low urinary output other than obstruction of the Foley catheter?

Yes. Bilateral ureteral obstruction (which is rare) can be monitored with ultrasound. Increased intra-abdominal pressure, which will cut off urinary output, must also be considered. This can be measured by transducing 50 ml of saline instilled through the Foley into the bladder. An intra-abdominal pressure greater than 30 mm Hg is incompatible with normal urinary function, and this pressure must be relieved in some way. Frequently the pressure is due to ascites, blood, or gas in the bowel, all of which may need to be evacuated in one way or another.

What should be done when the patient seems to be total body fluid overloaded, yet intravascularly depleted, and is oliguric?

Consider low-dose dopamine for the kidney and/or low-dose dobutamine for the heart. In addition, consider giving colloid to increase oncotic pressure in the blood. Gentle yet sustained diuresis to maintain a constant flow of urine out of the body and minimized fluid administration may also be helpful. Under these conditions one should be sure that there is always more out than in during each shift.

What is the single best parameter to determine a patient's overall fluid status?

Total body weight over time, especially when there is a preoperative weight available (which in theory shows the patient's normal weight)

How can a Foley that is suspected of malfunctioning be assessed?

The Foley can be flushed under sterile conditions with a Toomy syringe and sterile saline. If there is not free flow of this saline in and out of the Foley, the Foley should be changed.

What renal issues could arise that would kill your patient in the next 24 hours, and what can you do to lessen the likelihood of these issues arising?

Probably no renal issue can kill your patient in a day or less, but beware of the potential for lethal hyperkalemia in a patient with acute or chronic renal failure.

12

Gastrointestinal System

What are some GI health maintenance issues for the critically ill patient?

1. It's good to have food everywhere in the gut distal to the pylorus and very little food proximal to it.
2. Neutralize acid in the stomach or prevent its production.
3. Minimize the risk of aspiration.
4. Instill nystatin three to four times/day if the patient is taking antibiotics.
5. Follow the gallbladder with ultrasound if the right upper quadrant is tender, bilirubin level increases, or if occult fever occurs.
6. Monitor loose stool for *Clostridium difficile* colitis.

What GI issues could arise that would kill your patient in the next 24 hours, and what can you do to lessen the likelihood of these issues arising?

1. Aspiration pneumonitis. Keep the stomach decompressed. Always doubt that long, soft feeding tubes are in the small bowel—they are often in the stomach, or believe it or not, in the esophagus, pharynx, or airway. Don't resume oral feedings until the upper aerodigestive tract is working well.
2. Hemorrhage. Prevent gastritis by preventing gastric acid secretion or by neutralizing it. Be vigilant about occult GI bleeding.
3. Mesenteric ischemia. Have a low threshold for arteriogram. Watch lactic acid levels. Consider colonic ischemia if the patient has a bloody bowel movement, especially early after aortic aneurysm repair.
4. Bowel perforation. Have a low threshold for taking abdominal films. Decompress the colon if massively dilated (cecum larger than 10–12 cm). Keep the bowel decompressed (tubes), and watch what you're putting in if the bowel doesn't work well.

What are "herald bleeds?"

Episodes of bleeding in certain clinical situations that are mild in nature but predictive of more dangerous bleeding in the near future. (Remember that "bleed" is a verb, not a noun. When speaking or writing formally, use "hemorrhage" rather than bleed.)

Give two examples of herald bleeds.

1. Blood in a patient's tracheostomy tube representing partial erosion of the tube into the wall of the innominate artery. Emergent treatment if the artery is eroded includes inserting a finger into the stoma and compressing the artery against the underside of the sternum, after reintubation with a standard endotracheal tube.
2. Heme positive or grossly bloody stools in a patient with a history of abdominal aortic graft in place may represent erosion of the aortic graft into the duodenum. However, this complication is quite rare and responsible for only about 2% of GI bleeding in patients with aortic grafts.

What are "stress ulcers"?

Stress ulcer is the term used to describe the shallow, well-circumscribed mucosal erosions that can occur in the stomach and duodenum of seriously ill patients under extreme physiologic stress.

What factors predispose to stress ulcers?

1. Shock/hypotension
2. Sepsis
3. Burns (Curling's ulcers)
4. CNS trauma or tumor (Cushing's ulcers)

What causes stress ulcers?

The etiology is not entirely clear but is theorized to be initial mucosal injury secondary to ischemia and/or circulating toxins compounded by inadequate mucosal repair.

How do stress ulcers present?

Bleeding is the most frequent mode of presentation and can be occult or massive. Pain is an infrequent complaint.

What is the treatment for stress ulcers?

Most commonly, stress ulcers respond to antacids, H_2-blockers, and/or endoscopic therapy. Infusion of vasopressin into the left gastric artery has been used. Surgical therapy consists of either vagotomy, pyloroplasty, and suturing of bleeding points or vagotomy with subtotal gastrectomy. Total gastrectomy is rarely needed.

Can stress ulcers be prevented?

Yes. In most cases, prophylactic treatment of seriously ill patients with H_2-blockers is adequate.

Your patient develops a sinus tachycardia and then passes a large, maroon stool. What action should you take?

Secure good IV access and start fluid resuscitation. Catheters of short length and large gauge flow most rapidly. A peripheral 14-gauge, 5-cm catheter will flow much faster than a 16-gauge central venous pressure (CVP) catheter that may be more than 30 cm long.

In addition to frequent measurements of vital signs, what laboratory data should be obtained to assess the patient in the above question?

Check hemoglobin and be sure you have recent measurements of prothrombin time (PT), partial thromboplastin time (PTT), and platelet count. Type and cross match for at least 2 units of packed red blood cells.

In the situation presented, would you expect the hemoglobin to be higher, about the same, or lower than the day before?

About the same, at least until significant fluid resuscitation has occurred, producing a dilutional anemia from exogenously administered fluid, as well as the phenomenon of transcapillary refill

Define upper GI bleeding and lower GI bleeding.

1. Upper GI bleeding is bleeding between the lips and the ligament of Treitz.
2. Lower GI bleeding is bleeding from the ligament of Treitz to the anus. Most lower GI bleeding occurs in the colon, rectum, or anus.

Other than patient history, how can one gain valuable information within 5 minutes about the source of blood in the stool in an ICU patient?

Anorectal exam looking for bleeding hemorrhoids and gastric aspiration looking for blood to suggest an upper GI source

What is the best way to rule out or identify an upper GI source of bleeding?

Upper endoscopy, preceded by gastric lavage if needed

What is stress gastritis?

Multiple superficial erosions of the gastric mucosa

When does it occur?

It is common in any ICU setting, particularly in a patient "stressed" by severe acute illness, such as sepsis, shock, respiratory failure, and burns.

How often does it occur?

Endoscopic studies show that $2/3$–$3/4$ of critically ill patients in the ICU have endoscopic evidence of stress gastritis.

What is the pathogenesis?

Although some gastric acid is necessary, the primary cause is probably a decrease in the gastric mucosa's defense mechanisms against this acid, rather than increased acid production. Decreased defense mechanisms may be due to gastric mucosal hypoperfusion and ischemia.

How can it be prevented?

Reduction in intraluminal acid, which is accomplished equally well by H_2-blocker administration or liquid antacid use, is the mainstay of prevention.

How can adequate therapy be ensured?

With the use of H_2-blockers or antacids. The pH of the gastric aspirate must be tested to assess adequate therapy (pH > 5).

Is there any other type of therapy?

Sucralfate, which protects the mucosa by physically coating it, has been shown to be effective as well. The newer class of proton pump inhibitors, such as omeprazole, are extremely effective.

Which therapy is better?

There is no clear evidence that H_2-blockers, antacid therapy, or sucralfate is more efficacious than any therapy, but omeprazole may actually be superior to the others.

Who should get stress gastritis prophylaxis?

All critically ill patients in the ICU should have stress gastritis prophylaxis with one of the previously mentioned agents.

What is the most common complication of stress gastritis?

Bleeding

How should bleeding stress gastritis be initially treated?

1. Fluid resuscitation
2. Blood transfusion
3. Treatment of coagulopathy
4. Antacid therapy
5. NG suction
6. H_2-blockers

Initially, gastric lavage should be performed to remove the clot that contains fibrinolytic factors and increase stomach pH acutely. Correction of coagulopathy is another important early step.

Does endoscopy have a role?

Most patients treated with lavage and correction of coagulopathy will stop bleeding. Others may be helped by treating a localized area of bleeding with endoscopic electrocoagulation.

Which patients require surgery?

Patients who continue to manifest life-threatening bleeding from stress gastritis despite aggressive medical therapy and endoscopy. In patients bleeding from diffuse gastritis, this may require a total gastrectomy.

What disaster should you consider if your patient has a bowel movement in the first 24 hours after a major operation?

Colonic ischemia. If stool is bloody, this diagnosis is almost certain.

How can this diagnosis be confirmed?

Flexible lower GI endoscopy

How should it be treated?

Usually requires resection of sigmoid and left colon

In what order do the small bowel, large bowel, and stomach regain their activity after a period of ileus?

1. Small bowel function returns first (within 8 hours after surgery).
2. Colon function returns second (within 24–48 hours; slightly later return of lower GI activity with flatus and bowel movements).
3. Stomach function returns last (within 3–5 days; this late return may lead to devastating aspiration when the team is tricked into allowing food or fluid into the stomach too early).

How can gastric dilatation be detected?

1. Tympanitic left upper quadrant (check every day)
2. Large gastric air bubble on chest x-ray or on an abdominal x-ray [kidneys, ureter, bladder (KUB)]
3. Patient will be nauseated or at least anorectic if stomach is distended.

How can you keep the stomach empty in a critically ill patient?

1. Nasogastric suction
2. Keep nasogastric tube cleared by incessant attention to flushing with air and water.
3. Be absolutely certain that feeding tubes are not filling up the stomach.
4. Consider using metoclopramide (Reglan).
5. Don't assume the stomach works just because there are bowel sounds.
6. A poorly emptying stomach will drain better if the head of the bed is elevated.
7. Treat intra-abdominal inflammation.
8. Don't feed the patient until he or she is ready to eat.
9. Lobby for a jejunotomy tube if patient goes to OR for other procedures.

How can the GI tract quickly kill your patient?

1. Massive hemorrhage
2. Aspiration (Mendelson's syndrome)

How can the likelihood of these GI catastrophes be minimized?

1. Stress ulcer prophylaxis
2. Monitoring for lower GI hemorrhage
3. Keeping the stomach empty (except for antacids) until both your patient's mind and GI tract work

ACUTE ABDOMEN AND ABDOMINAL PAIN

What is the definition of acute abdomen?

An acute illness characterized by abdominal pain as the principal symptom in which early diagnosis and treatment are important. Treatment may be surgical or nonsurgical.

What are the types of abdominal pain?

Visceral, somatic, and referred

What are the characteristics of each?

1. Visceral afferents travel from irritated or stretched viscera with autonomic fibers via the splanchnic nerves to the spinal cord. Characterized by a vague, dull ache, or cramp located deep within the abdomen, making localization to a specific area difficult.
2. Somatic pain is derived from somatic innervation (spinal nerve fibers) of the abdominal wall and skin. More focused, intense, and constant than visceral pain. Results from irritation of the parietal peritoneum, thus making it easier to localize.
3. Referred pain is felt at a site distant to the disease, due to misinterpretation of a pain impulse traveling in an afferent fiber where multiple afferent fibers converge in the spinal cord (a shared central pathway).

Visceral pain is derived from the embryologic origin of which organs when referred to:

    The epigastrium?

Foregut: stomach, duodenum, biliary tract and pancreas

    Periumbilical?

Midgut: small intestine, right and transverse colon

    The hypogastrium?

Hindgut: distal transverse, descending, sigmoid colon, and rectum

What are the typical locations of referred pain from:	
Cholecystitis?	Right subscapular region
Diaphragmatic irritation?	Ipsilateral shoulder. When on the left, it's called Kehr's sign (subphrenic abscess, splenic injury)
Pancreatitis or pancreatic carcinoma?	Midback
Appendicitis?	Periumbilical early, right left quadrant, usually late
Rectal or uterine disease?	Low back
Nephrolithiasis or ureterolithiasis?	Ipsilateral flank or testicle
Ruptured aortic aneurysm?	Flank, back
What type of pain is usually the earliest indication of abdominal disease?	Visceral
Does this usually suggest that surgical intervention will be needed?	No. Visceral pain can come from many nonsurgical GI conditions, such as gastroenteritis.
What stimuli produce visceral pain?	1. Stretching of the wall of a hollow viscus or its mesentery by distension or contractions 2. Stretching of the capsule of a solid organ 3. Ischemia or inflammation within viscera
What type of pain usually suggests progressing or later intra-abdominal disease?	Somatic

Does this type of pain usually require surgical intervention?

Generally, if a visceral pain progresses to somatic pain, the need for surgical intervention is more likely.

What are the most helpful features in diagnosing the acute abdomen?

History and physical exam

What features of abdominal pain are important for diagnosis?

1. Location (local or referred)
2. Type (visceral or parietal)
3. Onset (seconds, minutes, hours)
4. Severity
5. Character (steady, intermittent, crampy, sharp, dull)
6. Factors that initiate or relieve the pain

What is peritonitis?

Inflammation of the peritoneum

What are the two major types of peritonitis?

1. Chemical (e.g., gastric acid, bile, barium, stool)
2. Infectious (inflammatory exudate)

What are peritoneal signs?

Findings on physical exam suggestive of peritonitis

What are these findings?

1. A patient lying still in bed, knees flexed with shallow respirations
2. Localized tenderness
3. Rebound and referred tenderness
4. Pain with any maneuver causing motion of the viscera within the peritoneal cavity
5. Voluntary guarding, involuntary guarding/rigidity

Most useful imaging studies?

Plain supine and erect radiographs, ultrasound, CT scan

Important common causes of abdominal pain in the ICU patient?

1. Gastritis, gastric/duodenal ulcer, ulcer perforation
2. Cholecystitis (calculous or acalculous, cholangitis)
3. Hepatitis
4. Pancreatitis
5. Bowel obstruction, mesenteric ischemia
6. Appendicitis, neutropenic enterocolitis

7. Colitis (ulcerative, bacterial, ischemic)
8. Intra-abdominal hemorrhage, spontaneous (abdominal aortic aneurysm rupture) or postoperative
9. Peritonitis from any of the above, anastomotic leak

Is the diagnosis of acute abdominal pain in the ICU patient more difficult?

YES! If you don't think about it, suspect it, and look for the subtle findings, you will miss it and the patient may die.

Why?

The history is often difficult or impossible to get (patient may be intubated, comatose, delirious). The exam is often altered and subtle.

What alters the physical exam?

1. Age. The elderly often have severe disease with minimal findings.
2. Altered pain perception (e.g., a distracting injury [a fresh incision], pain medications, altered sensorium, paraplegia/quadriplegia)
3. Impaired host defense. Malnutrition and immunosuppression cause inability to mount an inflammatory response.

GASTROINTESTINAL SYMPTOMS AND DYSFUNCTION

Where in the brain is food intake regulated?

In two areas of the hypothalamus: a lateral "feeding center" and a ventromedial "satiety center," which inhibits the feeding center, leading to satiety

What is anorexia?

The lack of desire to eat

Is it specific for abdominal disease?

No. Intra-abdominal inflammation, carcinoma, systemic disease, endocrinopathies, and drugs can all cause anorexia.

Is the absence of anorexia helpful in the diagnosis of acute abdominal disease?

Yes. The desire to eat generally suggests that the GI tract is ready to accept food or that a significant intra-abdominal pathologic condition is not present. The presence of hunger in a patient being worked up for appendicitis casts serious doubt on this diagnosis.

What is the treatment for anorexia?
Treat the inciting cause. No medications consistently stimulate appetite.

Definition of dysphagia?
Difficulty swallowing

Definition of odynophagia?
Painful swallowing

Swallowing is divided into what three stages?
Oral, pharyngeal, and esophageal

Airway protection occurs during which phase?
The pharyngeal

What is the mechanism for this?
The larynx and trachea are pulled superiorly by the suprahyoid muscles; the vocal cords close; and the epiglottis is displaced posteriorly.

From what does failure of this mechanism in ICU patients commonly result?
Altered mental status and tubes crossing this area interfere with its proper functioning. Inappropriate bed positioning (flat) also facilitates failure.

What are two major categories of dysphagia?
Oropharyngeal and esophageal

What are frequent causes of oropharyngeal dysphagia in the ICU patient?
1. Odynophagia (mucositis from chemotherapy/drugs, herpetic, fungal, or other mucosal lesions; pharyngitis [infectious or tube trauma])
2. Neuromuscular (head injuries, altered mental status)
3. Trauma to the face/neck

Frequent causes of esophageal dysphagia?
Most commonly due to luminal encroachment, but this is infrequently acute unless it is a result of surgery. Acute esophageal dysphagia is usually infectious (continuous, herpetic, fungal) or from direct trauma (including tubes).

Treatment of dysphagia?
First treat the cause: remove tubes/drugs, treat infections, repair injuries. Neurologic causes may require training to relearn swallowing. Once the cause is treated, topical treatment to relieve pain is often helpful.

What is nausea?	A feeling of the need to vomit
Does nausea always represent an intra-abdominal process?	Often, but not always. Its presence must be correlated to the clinical setting. Other causes include autonomic activation, drugs, uremia, radiation, and emotional disturbances.
What area of the brain mediates nausea?	Although not exactly known, evidence suggests it is similar to that described for vomiting (following).
What is treatment for nausea?	1. Treat the inciting cause. 2. Drugs: antihistamines, anticholinergics, phenothiazines, and dopaminergic antagonists
Are nausea and vomiting always linked?	No
What is vomiting?	The forceful expulsion of material from the GI tract through the mouth
Does vomiting always represent an intra-abdominal process?	No (see previous discussion of nausea)
Where is vomiting mediated in the brain?	The medulla
What are the two centers that regulate vomiting?	1. Chemoreceptor trigger zone (area postrema). Responsive to chemical stimuli in the circulation, but not electrical stimuli (afferent impulses). Requires an intact vomiting center to induce emesis. Function can be blocked by dopamine antagonists. 2. Vomiting center. Responsive to visceral afferent impulses (mucosal irritation, hollow viscus distension).
How is the act of vomiting coordinated?	The medulla initiates vomiting and coordinates the respiratory, truncal, and GI musculature to cause the forceful expulsion of GI contents while protecting the airway.

Does the pattern or character of the emesis help in diagnosis?

Yes

What diagnosis is suggested by the following patterns/characteristics of vomiting?

Immediately upon waking in the morning?

Increased intracranial pressure, pregnancy

Not preceded by nausea?

Increased intracranial pressure

Sudden and projectile?

Increased intracranial pressure

Repetitive, small volumes?

Toxins: food poisoning, gastroenteritis, drugs

Repetitive, large volumes, partially digested food?

Gastric outlet obstruction

Feculent?

Distal bowel obstruction, long-standing bowel obstruction, gastrocolic fistula

What is the typical fluid and electrolyte disturbance caused by persistent vomiting from gastric outlet obstruction?

Hypokalemic, hypochloremic metabolic alkalosis with volume depletion

If measured, what would the urinary pH be?

Acidic. Called paradoxical aciduria, it results in worsening of the metabolic alkalosis. Potassium and hydrogen ions are excreted to allow sodium conservation to counteract depleted circulating volume.

How should this condition be treated?

Volume repletion with intravenous normal saline and potassium

What is the treatment for vomiting?

1. Treatment of underlying cause
2. NG tube suctioning if appropriate
3. Drugs listed previously for the treatment of nausea, plus cisapride (prokinetic agent) or odansetron (5-HT_3 antagonist)
4. Aspiration precautions (e.g., elevate head of bed)

After a meal, the normal stomach empties within what amount of time?	Three to four hours
Complete passage of this food into the cecum requires how many hours?	Approximately 9 hours
Why is intestinal transit frequently delayed in ICU patients?	Intra-abdominal inflammation, metabolic disturbances, postoperative ileus, drugs (narcotics, anticholinergics)
Where is most of the water absorbed from the semiliquid chyme entering the colon?	In the cecum and ascending colon
Where is stool stored before defecation?	Sigmoid colon. It only passes into the rectum when defecation is about to occur.
Normal stool weight of an adult human per day?	About 200 g
Water accounts for what percentage of this weight?	About 80%
Definition of diarrhea?	Stool weights greater than 200 g/day. Typically described as greater stool frequency and liquidity.
What are the major pathophysiologic mechanisms of diarrhea?	Osmotic, secretory, inflammatory, and altered bowel motility. The common underlying defect is in intestinal water and electrolyte transport. This results in bowel distension, which stimulates peristalsis. The increased motility is thus usually secondary, not primary, in diarrhea.
The most common types in ICU patients?	Osmotic, inflammatory, secretory, or combinations of these
The general cause of osmotic diarrhea?	A non- or partially absorbed, orally ingested substance, which exerts an osmotic force, drawing fluid into the intestinal lumen

Typical features of osmotic diarrhea?

Diarrhea ceases on cessation of oral intake. Measured fecal osmolality is greater than calculated fecal osmolality (increased fecal osmotic gap).

Common specific causes of osmotic diarrhea in the ICU?

Drugs (lactulose) and enteral feeding

The general cause of inflammatory diarrhea?

Epithelial damage, mucosal and submucosal inflammation, loss of absorptive colonocytes

Typical features of inflammatory diarrhea?

Blood and leukocytes in the stool, inflammatory lesion on intestinal biopsy. Diarrhea persists with fasting. Patients frequently have fever, abdominal pain, and leukocytosis.

Common specific causes of inflammatory diarrhea in the ICU?

Drugs, infections (especially *Clostridium difficile*), and ischemia

The general mechanism of secretory diarrhea?

Active ion secretion by the intestinal epithelium with the passive movement of water into the intestinal lumen

Typical features of secretory diarrhea?

Large volumes, usually watery diarrhea. Fecal osmolality is isotonic (no fecal osmotic gap). Diarrhea is unaffected by fasting.

Common specific causes of secretory diarrhea in the ICU?

Drugs, infections

Most important initial part of the work-up for diarrhea in the ICU?

Take a history regarding drugs, recent antibiotic use, recent initiation of enteral feeds, period of hypotension (intestinal ischemia).

Most useful initial laboratory test for the work-up of diarrhea?

Microscopic examination of fresh stool for occult blood and leukocytes

The following findings on stool smear suggest which diagnosis?

1. RBCs and WBCs?

Inflammation with exudate (inflammatory bowel disease, invasive infection, *C. difficile* enterocolitis)

Next step in work-up?

Sigmoidoscopy/colonoscopy, stool for ova, parasites, and culture

2. RBCs, no WBCs?

Epithelial damage, no exudate (drugs, ischemia, neoplasm, *C. difficile*)

Next step in work-up?

Sigmoidoscopy/colonscopy, stool for *C. difficile* culture and toxin

3. No RBCs, no WBCs?

Osmotic or secretory diarrhea (drugs, enteral feeds, infection)

Next step in work-up?

Determine fecal osmolality and fecal osmotic gap, which help distinguish osmotic from secretory diarrhea.

Measured fecal osmolality normally approximates the osmolality of which body fluid?

Plasma (290 mOsm/L)

How is fecal osmolality calculated?

The sum of measured fecal Na^+ and K^+ multiplied by two (to account for anions)

How is fecal osmotic gap calculated?

Measured fecal osmolality minus calculated fecal osmolality

A fecal osmotic gap greater than 50 mOsm/L is typical of which type of diarrhea?

Osmotic. Secretory diarrhea osmolality is close to that of plasma.

How would you treat the following types of diarrhea?

1. Ischemic?

1. Restore circulating volume and perfusion, otherwise supportive unless complications supervene.

2. Infectious?

2. In the ICU patient, this is almost always *C. difficile* colitis, which is discussed following.

3. Osmotic?

3. In the ICU, this is usually a drug or enteral feedings. The drug should be stopped if possible; manipulation of enteral feedings is discussed in the nutrition section.

Is most antibiotic-associated diarrhea caused by an infection?

No. Most cases appear to be caused by an alteration in intestinal flora, not a specific infection.

How often is antibiotic-associated diarrhea complicated by infectious colitis?

About 10% of the time. *C. difficile* causes almost all of the cases.

How is *C. difficile* colitis treated?

1. Oral metronidazole
2. Oral vancomycin
3. IV metronidazole

13

Obstetrics and Gynecology

What are some gynecologic health maintenance issues in the female ICU patient?

1. Prescribe antifungal vaginal suppositories if patient is at risk for candidiasis (immunosuppression, broad-spectrum antibiotics, diabetes).
2. Use Nystatin powder liberally for groin and intertriginous folds.

Define preeclampsia and eclampsia.

1. Preeclampsia is the development of hypertension, albuminuria, and/or edema between the 20th week of pregnancy and the end of the first week postpartum.
2. Eclampsia is the above, plus coma and/or convulsions in the same time period without other etiology.

What are the incidences of each and the characteristics of the typical patient who develops preeclampsia?

Preeclampsia occurs in 5% of pregnancies, typically in primigravidas with preexisting hypertension or vascular disease. If untreated, preeclampsia typically smolders for a variable length of time, then suddenly progresses to eclampsia. Eclampsia develops in 1 in 200 preeclamptic patients and is usually fatal if untreated.

What are the guidelines for diagnosis of preeclampsia?

Any pregnant patient who develops a blood pressure (BP) greater than 140/90 or has an increase in BP of 30 mm Hg systolic or 15 mm Hg diastolic, edema of the face or hands, or albuminuria of 1+ or more.

Differentiate between mild and severe preeclampsia.

Mild preeclampsia is considered to be borderline hypertension, mild edema, or mild albuminuria. Preeclampsia is considered severe if BP is greater than 150/110 or if edema and albuminuria are marked.

Outline the treatment of preeclampsia.

Mild preeclampsia may respond to strict bed rest. If it does not respond within 48 hours of bed rest, hospitalization is indicated. Severe preeclampsia is treated with IV $MgSO_4$ until hyperreflexia and hypertension improve. Additional antihypertensive therapy is occasionally needed, as is diuretic therapy. After 32–34 weeks' gestation, fetal maturity should be assessed and prompt delivery of the infant undertaken when maturity is assured.

Eclampsia is also treated with IV $MgSO_4$ until seizures respond. Supplementation with IV diazepam may be required. Delivery of the fetus should be accomplished as soon as the mother is stabilized.

OBSTETRIC SHOCK

Define shock.

Shock can be defined simply as inadequate tissue perfusion.

What is the most common cause of hypovolemic shock in obstetrics and what are the conditions that cause it?

Hemorrhage (abruptio placentae, placenta previa, placenta accreta, retained products of conception, uterine atony or rupture, obstetric lacerations, surgical procedures)

What volume of blood loss should alert you to the possibility of significant postpartum bleeding?

More than 500 ml

What fraction of maternal blood volume can be lost before hypotension and inadequate tissue perfusion ensue?

One-fourth of maternal blood volume (class II shock)

What maternal lab values correlate with fetal distress?

Decreased maternal serum bicarbonate and increased lactic acid levels

What measures can be taken to decrease postpartum uterine bleeding?

1. Uterine massage
2. Oxytocin IV
3. Intravaginal prostaglandin E_2. If examination of the placenta reveals fragmentation, the uterus must be manually examined for retained products. Persistent bleeding may require hysterectomy.

What are the common obstetric conditions leading to septic shock in obstetric patients?

1. Antepartum pyelonephritis
2. Septic abortion
3. Chorioamnionitis
4. Postpartum endometritis

Outline the clinical findings that should prompt the investigation for postpartum infection.

Even in the first 12 hours, a significant fever must be evaluated by examination of the lungs and uterus, and cultures of the urine and lochia. Puerperal infection must be assumed if the patient has a temperature greater than 38°C on two successive days following the first 24 hours and other causes have been excluded. With progression, tachycardia and leukocytosis develop, and the uterus is commonly enlarged, soft, and tender.

What conditions predispose the patient to postpartum infection?

Anemia, preeclampsia, prolonged rupture of the membranes, prolonged labor, traumatic delivery, repeated examinations, retention of placental fragments, and postpartum hemorrhage

Name the single most common bacterial pathogen isolated in obstetrical sepsis.

Escherichia coli is isolated in one-fourth to one-half of all cases.

What other organisms are frequently present in obstetrical sepsis?

Staphylococci, β-hemolytic *Streptococcus,* anaerobic streptococci, enteric gram-negative organisms, *Enterococcus,* and *Clostridium perfringens.*

What empiric antibiotic therapy is indicated in obstetrical sepsis?

"Triple coverage," i.e., a regimen providing coverage against aerobic *Streptococcus, Staphylococcus,* enteric gram-negative organisms, and anaerobes. The gold standard in the past has been ampicillin, gentamicin, and clindamycin, although many different combinations provide adequate coverage.

TRAUMA AND PREGNANCY

What are the normal physiologic changes that occur during pregnancy in each of the following:

Cardiac output?

Increases ≈ 1.5 L/min

Heart rate?

Increases ≈ 15 beats/min

Blood pressure?

Decreases ≈ 15 mm Hg during second trimester and returns to normal by delivery

EKG?

1. Left axis deviation
2. Flattened or inverted T waves in III, AVF, and precordial leads
3. Increased ectopy

Blood volume?

Increases by one-half

White blood cell (WBC) count?

Can increase to 20,000

PCO_2?

Decreases to ≈ 30 mm Hg late in pregnancy

Gastric emptying?

Very delayed; stomach must be considered full at all times.

Pituitary gland?

May double in weight and may undergo necrosis during periods of shock (Sheehan's syndrome)

Neurologic?

Seizures and hyperreflexia; think eclampsia (with or without hypertension).

How should you position the pregnant trauma patient?

On her left side, if possible. If spine injury is present or during CPR, the right hip should be elevated and the uterus manually retracted to the left.

Why?	The uterus compresses the vena cava, causing venous hypertension in the lower extremities and reducing cardiac output by one-third.
Do a normal pulse, BP, and PO₂ predict adequate resuscitation to protect the fetus?	No
Why?	Uterine blood flow is very sensitive to catecholamines and may be reduced by one-fourth without any change in maternal BP.
What approach should be taken for the "minimally" injured pregnant patient?	All patients should be given liberal fluid resuscitation and supplemental oxygen. Consult the Ob/Gyn service for all patients and for fetal heart monitoring.
What test should be used to rule out intra-abdominal injury: CT or diagnostic peritoneal lavage (DPL)?	DPL. This test has been shown to be safe in the pregnant patient. A supraumbilical, open approach should be used. CT has the disadvantages of exposing the fetus to radiation, of being time consuming, and of missing a significant percentage of hollow viscus injuries.
What is the rate of placental abruption from blunt trauma?	5% of "minor" injuries and up to one-half of major injuries
What are the common findings with placental abruption?	Uterine tenderness, vaginal bleeding, uterine contractions, fetal distress. Some patients exhibit no pain or bleeding, making uterine and fetal monitoring mandatory.

OTHER OB/GYN COMPLICATIONS

What is HELLP syndrome?	**H**emolysis **E**levated **L**iver enzymes **L**ow **P**latelets in a patient with preeclampsia

What is the differential diagnosis of third-trimester bleeding?	Placenta previa, abruption, fetal hemorrhage
Common causes of postpartum hemorrhage?	Uterine atony, retained placenta, vaginal or cervical laceration
What is placental abruption?	Premature separation of the placenta from the uterus
What are the main complications of abruption?	Hemorrhage, disseminated intravascular coagulopathy (DIC), and fetal death
What are the different types and the significance of fetal heart rate decelerations?	Early, head compression; variable, cord compression; late, uteroplacental insufficiency
What is the significance of a sinusoidal fetal heart rate pattern?	Severe fetal anemia or hypoxia
What is an ectopic pregnancy?	A conceptus that is implanted outside the uterus
What are the potential complications of an ectopic pregnancy?	Rupture, hemorrhage, and maternal death
What clinical parameters indicate a suspicion for ectopic pregnancy?	Last menstrual period more than 4 weeks, lower abdominal pain, vaginal bleeding, +/- unilateral mass on pelvic exam, nonclotting blood on culdocentesis
How do you make the definitive diagnosis of an ectopic pregnancy?	Quantitative β-hCG > 2000 and no intrauterine pregnancy (IUP) on transvaginal ultrasound (TV US), or quantitative β-hCG > 6000 and no IUP on transabdominal (TA) US.
What is necrotizing fasciitis?	A rapidly advancing and lethal bacterial infection in which there is necrosis of skin and subcutaneous tissue
Which gynecologic patients are at highest risk?	Diabetics with a Bartholin's gland abscess

| **How do you manage these patients?** | Stabilize rapidly—give electrolytes, hydrate, and cross-match multiple units of blood, and immediately take to the OR for extensive debridement of skin, subcutaneous fat, and +/– fascia. Involve Plastic Surgery because of the extensive tissue removal. |

AMNIOTIC FLUID EMBOLISM

Is amniotic fluid embolism (AFE) common?	No, it's rare. The incidence in the U.S. is 1:50,000 live births.
What are the signs and symptoms of an AFE?	Acute shortness of breath, hypoxia, and shock, followed by mental status changes, hemorrhage, and DIC
Which patients are at high risk for AFE?	Patients with an intrauterine fetal demise (IUFD); those taking oxytocin; and those with a short, abrupt course of labor.
When should AFE be suspected?	Whenever sudden, unexplained peripartum respiratory distress, hypotension, pulmonary edema, or coagulopathy develops.
What are the common and uncommon symptoms?	1. One-half of patients develop respiratory distress and cyanosis. 2. One-fourth develop hypotension. 3. One-fourth develop pulmonary edema. 4. Four in ten develop coagulopathy. 5. One in ten develops seizures. Bronchospasm and chest pain occur rarely in AFE, and their presence suggests pulmonary thromboembolism as a cause of symptoms.
What are the common diagnostic and laboratory findings?	1. Arterial blood gas indicates maternal hypoxemia. 2. Coagulopathy with prolonged clotting times and elevated fibrin split products with hypofibrinogenemia are found. 3. Chest x-ray findings are nonspecific, with pulmonary edema frequently noted.

4. ECG findings are also nonspecific with tachycardia, ST and T wave changes, and a pattern of right ventricular strain.

How is the diagnosis made?

Identification of amniotic debris in blood taken from the right side of the heart via a pulmonary artery catheter is diagnostic. Special stains assist in identifying such material.

What is the treatment for AFE?

Therapy is supportive. Hypoxemia is corrected with supplemental oxygen and frequently requires intubation and mechanical ventilation. Pulmonary artery catheterization and inotropic support should also be considered. Coagulopathy is corrected with fresh frozen plasma and cryoprecipitate. Low-dose heparin, aspirin, and antifibrinolytic agents may also be necessary, as in the treatment of DIC from other causes.

What is the prognosis?

Poor. The mortality rate remains between 75% and 90%.

DIC IN OBSTETRICS

What is DIC?

Disseminated intravascular coagulation, a pathologic condition associated with inappropriate activation of coagulation and fibrinolysis due to some underlying disease state.

What are the signs and symptoms of DIC?

Findings are variable but can include generalized hemorrhage, localized bleeding, purpura, petechiae, and thromboembolic phenomena. End-organ damage can result from intravascular fibrin deposits.

What laboratory abnormalities occur in DIC?

Thrombocytopenia, elevated prothrombin time (PT) and less often partial thromboplastin time (PTT), elevated thrombin time, elevation of D-dimer and fibrin split products, and a decline in fibrinogen.

What obstetric complications may be associated with DIC?	Abruptio placentae, fetal demise, preeclampsia/eclampsia, AFE, saline or septic abortion, sepsis

What is the treatment for DIC?

(Note: Some aspects remain controversial.)
1. Treat inciting disease process (sometimes all that is required).
2. Halt intravascular coagulation: low-dose subcutaneous or IV heparin (equally effective), antiplatelet agents (aspirin), antithrombin concentrates.
3. If patient is still bleeding after above measures, replace platelets (platelet concentrates) and clotting factors (fresh frozen plasma, cryoprecipitate) based on laboratory values.
4. Finally, consider inhibition of fibrinolysis (ε-aminocaproic acid or tranexamic acid) only if above measures have failed. These agents may precipitate fatal thromboses if patient is not anticoagulated first!

What is the prognosis?	Related to the underlying cause

THROMBOEMBOLIC DISEASE DURING PREGNANCY

What is the incidence of ante- and postpartum deep vein thrombosis (DVT) and pulmonary embolism (PE)?	The incidence of DVT in this population is estimated to be between 7 in 1000 and 1 in 2500. PE is estimated to be 1 in 2700 to 1 in 7000.
Is it a significant cause of maternal mortality?	PE causes 10%–15% of all maternal deaths.
Are pregnant women at a greater or lesser risk of developing a DVT than nonpregnant women?	Greater risk. Pregnant women are estimated to be five times more likely to develop a DVT.
What is the anatomic distribution of DVTs in pregnancy?	During pregnancy, thrombosis occurs in the pelvic veins more frequently than occurs in nonpregnant women and much more frequently in the left leg than in the right.

Why is the distribution different in pregnancy?

The gravid uterus places pressure on the inferior vena cava and iliac veins, thus creating stasis in the veins of the lower extremities. Because the inferior vena cava is normally to the right of midline, the left iliac vein has to cross over behind the left iliac artery and therefore is more prone to compression than is the right.

What is Virchow's triad?

Virchow postulated that venous thrombosis is related to three factors: 1) vessel endothelial injury, 2) vascular stasis, and 3) increased coagulability.

Are there any other predisposing factors in pregnancy?

Advanced maternal age, traumatic delivery, cesarean section, thrombophlebitis, and endometritis

How do you diagnose a DVT?

1. Venography is the gold standard but requires contrast and radiation and can itself induce venous thrombosis.
2. Real-time β-mode US is now most commonly used. However, US cannot reliably detect iliac, pelvic, or calf vessel thrombosis.
3. Impedance plethysmography also can be used but has generally been replaced by US.
4. MRI can reliably detect thrombosis of not only the femoral veins but also the pelvic veins. This option should be considered if US of the legs is negative and suspicion is high.

What are the most common symptoms and findings following a PE?

More than 80% of patients complain of chest pain and dyspnea; 90% will have a respiratory rate greater than 16 breaths/min. The PO_2 is almost always 60 or less, and the PCO_2 is almost always low.

What diagnostic tests are used to confirm a PE?

The extent to which one needs to confirm the presence of a PE is controversial.
1. The gold standard is a pulmonary arteriogram.
2. Ventilation–perfusion scintigraphy (V/Q scan) is now commonly used

and gives results as normal or low, medium, or high probability. High probability scans usually indicate a PE. However, many scans do not result in high probability scans and, in addition, this test's accuracy goes down significantly when there are ventilation defects from other lung diseases. If therapy will be altered by a positive result and clinical suspicion is high in the face of an indeterminate V/Q scan, proceed with an arteriogram. A normal scan with low clinical suspicion makes PE very unlikely.

What about radiation risks?

Each of these tests provides less than 50 mrad to the fetus if performed properly and should be obtained if clinically indicated.

What is the treatment for thromboembolic disease in pregnancy?

Treatment in the postpartum patient is the same as for nongravid patients.

- Antepartum thromboembolic disease requires special consideration. In general, heparin is safe and effective and does not cross the placental barrier. Intravenous heparin should be administered to keep the PTT 1.5–2.5 times normal. Heparin should be discontinued during active labor; it should be restarted within several hours of a normal delivery but should be delayed for 1–2 days if there is significant trauma to the lower genital tract.
- Warfarin is thought to be teratogenic in the first 8 weeks of pregnancy and may cross the placenta, placing the fetus at increased risk of hemorrhage and should therefore be avoided.
- Patients with a very recent PE and a need to be delivered by C-section should be considered for placement of a vena caval filter prior to surgery.
- Gravid patients who had a DVT during a previous pregnancy should be maintained on low-dose heparin throughout their pregnancy.

14

Endocrine System

What are some of the endocrinologic maintenance issues for the critically ill patient?

1. Be sure stress steroids are ordered if there is any chance of adrenal suppression.
2. Monitor glucose and have a very low threshold to use an insulin drip. [This can drive insulin into tissues where it's needed (e.g., the heart), can help treat acidosis, and can avoid confusing fluid status when significant glycosuria is present.]
3. Have a low threshold for checking thyroid function tests. Many ill patients are hypothyroid.

What endocrine issue could arise that would kill your patient in the next 24 hours, and what can you do to lessen the likelihood of this issue arising?

Hypoglycemia.
1. Ensure adequate glucose delivery.
2. Guard against reactive hypoglycemia (seen with sudden withdrawal of glucose).
3. Monitor glucose levels.
4. Don't control glucose too tightly. (Better too much glucose than too little!)

STRESS RESPONSE PHYSIOLOGY

Which of the following are increased, decreased, or unchanged during the "normal" stress response as would be observed in the ICU, and what is the overall physiologic effect?

This is really simple if you think about the "fight or flight" response and remember three basic concepts of stress response physiology:
- Maintenance of blood pressure
- Conservation of glucose for the brain
- Shift of metabolism toward catabolism of protein and fat

1. Catecholamines

Increased. Secreted from sympathetic nerve terminals and adrenal medulla, catecholamines are the main component of the "fight or flight" response. They help to maintain blood pressure by producing vasoconstriction (alpha) and increasing cardiac output (beta). The glucose available for the brain is increased by inhibition of insulin secretion (alpha) and stimulation of glucagon secretion (beta), gluconeogenesis, and glycogenolysis (beta). Metabolism is shifted to the peripheral catabolism of fat and protein.

2. Vasopressin (ADH)   Increased. Secreted from the posterior pituitary (neurohypophysis) in response to high serum osmolality, ADH is a potent vasoconstrictor and acts on the kidney to retain free water. Both of these functions serve to maintain blood pressure.

3. Renin   Increased. Stimulated by increased catecholamines, decreased renal perfusion, and decreased serum Na^+, juxtaglomerular apparatus cells in kidney release renin to preserve blood pressure. Renin converts plasma angiotensinogen to angiotensin I, followed by conversion to angiotensin II via angiotensin converting enzyme (ACE) in the lungs. Angiotensin II is a potent vasoconstrictor and stimulates aldosterone secretion, both of which serve to maintain blood pressure.

4. Aldosterone   Increased. Adrenal secretion is stimulated by decreased serum Na^+, increased K^+, adrenocorticotropic hormone (ACTH), and angiotensin II. Aldosterone maintains blood pressure by increasing blood volume, resulting in renal resorption of Na^+, and therefore H_2O, and loss of K^+.

5. ACTH/glucocorticoid (cortisone) axis   Increased. Cortisone makes more glucose available for the brain by increased peripheral gluconeogenesis and insulin resistance, which results in decreased peripheral glucose utilization. Also, this hormone shifts peripheral catabolism/ metabolism to fat and protein.

6. Insulin

Decreased/unchanged. This results in decreased peripheral glucose utilization, making more glucose available for the brain.

7. Glucagon

Increased. Increases the glucose available for the brain by increasing gluconeogenesis and glycolysis and shifts metabolism to catabolism of fat and protein

8. Growth hormone

Increased. Produces decreased glucose transport into cells and peripheral insulin resistance, which results in decreased glucose utilization, thus making more glucose available to the brain

9. Thyroid hormones

Decreased/unchanged. It was postulated that in critical stress states these should be elevated and that some of the pathophysiology of critical illness was due to inappropriate euthyroidism. This hypothesis led to use of the term "sick-euthyroid syndrome." Clinical trials have disproved this hypothesis, and a euthyroid or slightly hypothyroid state is normal pathophysiology for critical stress.

DYSREGULATION SYNDROMES

What is thyroid storm?

Severe hyperthyroidism manifesting as marked increases in T_3 and T_4, resulting in profound hypermetabolism and hyperpyrexia. Body temperatures may be so high that enzyme systems fail.

What is the treatment?

1. Cool with cooling blankets, intubate, and paralyze to stop the heat production of shivering.
2. Decrease thyroid hormone production with propylthiouracil or methimazole.
3. Decrease thyroid hormone release with iodides (Lugol's solution) or lithium.
4. Decrease thyroid hormone response by β-blockade with propranolol.

What is addisonian crisis and what are its clinical manifestations?

Adrenal insufficiency that manifests with fever, nausea/vomiting, abdominal pain, hypotension, and altered mental status due to glucocorticoid insufficiency. Mineralocorticoid (aldosterone) insufficiency results in hyponatremia and hypokalemia.

What is the most common etiology of addisonian crisis?

Inadvertent withdrawal of exogenous steroids and/or failure to provide "stress dose" steroids after suppression of endogenous glucocorticoid production by long-term administration of steroids.

What are "stress dose" steroids?

Dose of corticosteroids required to approximate the fourfold increase in production normally found during times of stress—usually hydrocortisone 100 mg q 8 hrs slowly tapered. This regimen will prevent or treat adrenal insufficiency.

What is SIADH?

Syndrome of inappropriate antidiuretic hormone release, which results in inappropriate retention of free water

What causes it?

Stress states (e.g., sepsis, infection, surgery, trauma), malignancy, brain trauma, or surgery

What are the clinical and lab findings?

Volume overload, edema, hyponatremia

How is it treated?

By restriction of free water intake and treatment of the underlying cause

A patient undergoes a routine pulmonary resection and receives 2800 ml of ½ normal saline. The patient has neither vomiting nor nasogastric suction. Serum sodium is 142 mEq/L before surgery. On the first postoperative day, sodium is 128 mEq/L. What hormonal response to the stress of surgery may have produced this dilutional hyponatremia?

Posterior pituitary produces an increased amount of ADH (antidiuretic hormone) in response to the stress of surgery. Thus, the body retains fluid and dilutes the sodium in the plasma.

15

Hematology

What are some hematologic health maintenance issues for the critically ill patient?

1. Deep venous thrombosis (DVT) prophylaxis (heparin, stockings, boots)
2. Aspirin (acetylsalicylic acid) for patients with atherosclerotic disease
3. Competence of coagulation system (vitamin K in total parenteral nutrition [TPN], monitor parameters)
4. Monitor platelet counts if on heparin (subcutaneous [SQ], therapeutic, or even flushes).
5. Monitor prothrombin time (PT) and international normalized ratio (INR) if on Coumadin.
6. Ensure platelet count greater than 50,000 for invasive procedures.
7. Monitor platelet count if receiving antilymphocyte therapy for immunosuppression induction.
8. When feasible, fully anticoagulate patients with atrial fibrillation, mechanical heart valves, DVT, or arterial emboli from heart.

What hematologic issues could arise that would kill your patient in the next 24 hours, and what can you do to lessen the likelihood of these issues arising?

1. Anemia:
   Transfuse prn.
   Monitor blood loss.
2. Venous thromboembolic disease:
   DVT prophylaxis
   Anticoagulate if clot is present intravascularly.
3. Heparin-associated thrombocytopenia and thrombosis (HATT) syndrome:
   Monitor platelets daily if on heparin.
   Suspect HATT if exposure to heparin has been prolonged or repeated and, with platelet count falling, evidence of thrombosis.
4. Disseminated intravascular coagulopathy (DIC):

Monitor coagulants.
Obtain fibrin split products if DIC is
  suspected.
Treat potential causes of DIC.
Suspect if odd bleeding patterns are
  evident.

**What measures can be
taken to prevent DVT in a
bedridden ICU patient?**

1. Low-dose heparin
2. Sequential compression stockings

**What is the first line of
treatment for DVT?**

Anticoagulation with heparin

**What is the purpose of
using heparin in cases of
DVT?**

To decrease the chance of pulmonary
embolism (PE) and to prevent clot
propagation

**What is the recommended
treatment for a patient
who presents with DVT
and PE, and then, after
anticoagulation, develops a
major bleeding problem?**

1. Stop the heparin and consider
   reversing its effect with Protamine.
2. Place a vena cava filter.

**What is the differential
diagnosis for eosinophilia?**

Remember the mnemonic **NAACP:**
Neoplasm
Addison's disease
Asthma and Allergic disease
Connective tissue disease
Parasite infection

**When a patient is
bleeding, what coagulation
deficits might be present
and how can they be
corrected?**

1. Exposed endothelium (i.e., open
   blood vessel):
   Operative Rx (Bovie, Prolene, etc.)
   Lower BP with nitroprusside.
2. Impaired intrinsic coagulation
   cascade:
   Reverse heparin with Protamine.
3. Impaired extrinsic coagulation
   cascade:
   Fresh frozen plasma
   IV vitamin K
4. Decreased fibrinogen:
   Cryoprecipitate
5. Increased fibrinolysis (after cardiac or
   thoracic surgery):
   ϵ-aminocaproic acid

6. Temperature under 37°C:
   Warm patient (hypothermia impairs clotting).
7. Decreased number or dysfunction of platelets:
   Desmopressin (DDAVP)
   Platelet transfusion
   Dialysis if uremic
   Discontinue drugs known to decrease platelet number or function.

What are the four phases of hemostasis?

1. Vascular phase (vasospasm)
2. Platelet plug phase (primary hemostasis)
3. Fibrin clot phase (secondary hemostasis)
4. Clot lysis phase (fibrinolysis)

What single disease process causes a defect in all four phases?

Cirrhosis:
1. Vascular phase: varices
2. Platelet plug phase: thrombocytopenia (splenomegaly)
3. Fibrin clot phase: decreased hepatic synthesis of clotting factors
4. Clot lysis phase: decreased hepatic clearance of fibrin split products

POSTSURGICAL BLEEDING AND BLOOD TRANSFUSIONS

What is the most common cause of excessive postsurgical bleeding?

Failure of local mechanical hemostasis (i.e., the "surgical bleeder," otherwise known as exposed endothelium)

What is the treatment?

Re-exploration and cautery or suturing

Other disorders of the vascular phase?

Infiltrative disorders (e.g., amyloidosis), inflammatory disorders (e.g., vasculitis), nutritional deficiencies (e.g., scurvy), varices, telangiectasias, hemangiomas, angiodysplasia

How do damaged blood vessels contribute to hemostasis?

Vascular spasm, expression of tissue factors and exposure of subendothelial collagen (both are potent procoagulants)

What are the causes of abnormal mediastinal bleeding after cardiopulmonary bypass (CPB)?

1. Failure of local mechanical hemostasis (i.e., an anatomic bleeder)
2. Pump-induced platelet dysfunction
3. The **three Hs: H**ypothermia (reversible platelet and clotting factor dysfunction), **H**emodilution (thrombocytopenia, decreased clotting factors), **H**eparin (inadequate reversal with Protamine, "heparin rebound")
4. Fibrinolysis

What is the most important cause of nonsurgical bleeding after CPB?

Platelet dysfunction

How much does 1 unit of packed red blood cells (PRBCs) raise the hematocrit (HCT)?

~ 3%

Characteristics of PRBCs?

1 unit = 250–350 ml, HCT = 50%–80%, stored at 1°C–6°C, citrate used as anticoagulant

What factors influence the decision to transfuse PRBCs?

Patient's age; severity of anemia; intravascular volume status; underlying heart, lung, or vascular disease

What is the minimum hemoglobin (Hgb) level tolerated by a normovolemic, healthy adult?

7 mg/dl (below this level, oxygen-carrying capacity is inadequate to sustain normal cardiopulmonary function)

What is the minimum Hgb tolerated by elderly patients with coronary artery disease?

10 mg/dl

What is the minimum Hgb tolerated by a critically ill patient with coronary artery disease?

10 mg/dl (keep hematocrit above 30)

What are the appropriate indications for blood transfusion?

1. The need to increase the concentration of RBCs to increase O_2 delivery
2. To increase clotting ability; giving functional platelets will facilitate clotting and stop bleeding
3. Volume resuscitation for hypovolemic shock

What should you remember at the bedside about giving blood?

1. Warm the blood product; cold blood will lower a patient's core body temp.
2. Add Ca^+ to avoid the complications of hypocalcemia (i.e., tetany and bleeding disorders). (The anticoagulants used in stored blood chelate Ca^{++}.)
3. Remember to give platelets every time 10 units of blood are given.

Potential complications of massive PRBC transfusion?

1. Hyperkalemia (efflux from RBCs)
2. Hypocalcemia (citrate is a calcium chelator)
3. Acid–base derangements (prolonged storage of blood promotes acidosis due to lactate production, or citrate can be metabolized to bicarbonate to produce alkalosis)
4. Dilutional thrombocytopenia
5. Disseminated intravascular coagulation
6. Increased affinity of Hgb for oxygen (decreased 2,3-DPG levels with prolonged storage, low temp, and alkalosis from citrate metabolism all conspire to shift oxy-Hgb curve to the left, thus decreasing release of O_2)
7. Systemic hypothermia (blood stored at 1°C–6°C)

What are some other adverse effects?

Transfusion reactions, viral transmissions

What is the frequency of transfusion reactions?

10%–15% of all patients receiving blood

What is the most common type?

Febrile reaction (characterized by fever, chills, flushing, and urticaria)

What causes a transfusion reaction?	Minor leukocyte antigens
What is the treatment?	Diphenhydramine if mild, epinephrine and/or corticosteroids if severe
Which is the most severe type?	Hemolytic transfusion reaction (1/6000)
What is the cause of a hemolytic transfusion reaction?	ABO incompatibility (most commonly a clerical error)

What are the clinical features of a hemolytic transfusion reaction?

1. Fever (earliest sign)
2. Anxiety/agitation
3. Flushing
4. Chest pain
5. Flank/back pain
6. Reddish discoloration of urine (hemoglobinuria)
7. DIC (release of thromboplastin)
8. Renal failure (pigment nephropathy)
9. Vascular collapse (release of vasoactive amines)

What is the treatment?

1. Stop transfusion immediately!
2. Insert urinary catheter.
3. Vigorous fluid resuscitation
4. Intravenous $NaHCO_3$ to alkalinize urine and thus mitigate effects of free Hgb on kidneys (pigment nephropathy)
5. Mannitol (osmotic diuresis)
6. Vasopressors (if necessary to support circulation)

What is the risk of viral transmission from 1 unit of blood?	HIV: 1/225,000 Hepatitis B: 1/200,000 Hepatitis C: 1/3300
What is the most common transfusion-associated hepatitis infection in the U.S.?	Hepatitis C
What is the most common bleeding disorder after a massive blood transfusion?	Dilutional thrombocytopenia

PLATELETS AND DISORDERS OF PRIMARY HEMOSTASIS

What are the two general classes of disorders of primary hemostasis?	1. Platelet dysfunction 2. Thrombocytopenia
Signs of primary hemostatic disorders?	Usually mild, superficial mucocutaneous bleeding that begins immediately after minor trauma or invasive procedure and is easily controlled; examples include: 1. Bleeding into skin (easy bruisability, petechiae, ecchymoses, purpura) 2. Bleeding after minor mucous membrane trauma/surgery (epistaxis) 3. Oozing from skin incisions or sites of percutaneous catheters
What is platelet dysfunction?	A qualitative defect in platelet adhesion, activation, secretion, or aggregation, regardless of the platelet count
What are the most common acquired causes of platelet dysfunction in the ICU patient?	1. Drugs = #1 cause! Especially aspirin (single most common cause of platelet dysfunction), other NSAIDs, β-lactam antibiotics, nitroglycerin, furosemide 2. Uremia (interference with von Willebrand factor [vWF]–mediated platelet adhesion) 3. Hypothermia (Cold blood doesn't clot!)
How does ASA affect platelets?	Irreversibly acetylates and inhibits the enzyme cyclo-oxygenase, thereby inhibiting thromboxane A_2 production and its platelet aggregatory effects
What is the onset of action of ASA?	2 hours
What is the duration of action of ASA?	7–9 days (entire life span of the platelet)
What is the lab test for diagnosis of platelet dysfunction?	Bleeding time (prolonged)

What is normal bleeding time?	Less than 5 minutes
How should one treat platelet dysfunction?	Depends on etiology: Drugs: discontinue offending agents, platelet transfusions for severe or persistent bleeding Uremia: dialysis, DDAVP, cryoprecipitate, conjugated estrogens Hypothermia: warming blankets/lights, warm fluids, and respiratory gases
Most common inherited causes of platelet dysfunction?	von Willebrand syndromes, which are also the most common group of serious inherited hemostatic disorders in general
What are von Willebrand syndromes?	Autosomal dominant disorders with multiple subtypes characterized by a qualitative or quantitative defect in vWF.
What are the lab tests for diagnosis of von Willebrand syndromes?	1. Prolonged bleeding time (low vWF) 2. Elevated partial thromboplastin time (PTT; low factor VIII:C activity)
What is the treatment for von Willebrand syndromes?	DDAVP (for type I only), cryoprecipitate, factor VIII concentrate (depends on subtype)
What is DDAVP?	1-deamino-8-D-arginine vasopressin or desmopressin; an antidiuretic hormone (ADH) analog with hemostatic properties (stimulates release of preformed vWF and factor VIII:C from endothelial cells)
How is DDAVP used in ICU patients?	1. To control clinically significant bleeding from acquired platelet dysfunction (especially uremia), type I von Willebrand syndrome, mild hemophilia A, and after cardiopulmonary bypass 2. Diabetes insipidus
What are the side effects of DDAVP?	Tachyphylaxis, hyponatremia, seizures

How is thrombocytopenia defined?

Usually a platelet count less than 100,000 is used to define thrombocytopenia, as the bleeding time is prolonged below this level.

What are the signs of thrombocytopenia?

The same as in other primary hemostatic disorders, except that spontaneous internal hemorrhage can occur with platelet counts below 20,000 (including lethal intracranial hemorrhage)

What are the common causes of thrombocytopenia in the ICU patient?

1. Decreased platelet production (marrow suppression) from: Drugs (H_2-blockers are very common offenders in the ICU) Sepsis
2. Platelet sequestration from splenomegaly, as in a patient with portal hypertension
3. Increased destruction as a result of: Immunologic destruction: drugs (heparin, quinidine, sulfa) and autoimmune disorders Increased utilization: DIC, sepsis, severe hemorrhage with massive blood transfusion Mechanical destruction: prosthetic cardiac valves, vascular prostheses, intra-aortic balloon pump
(Note: *Drugs* are the single most common cause of a deficit in platelet function or number!)

Lab test for diagnosis of thrombocytopenia?

Platelet count: 50,000–100,000 = minor; 20,000–50,000 = moderate; less than 20,000 = severe

What platelet count is considered adequate to safely undergo surgery or an invasive procedure?

50,000 or greater

Indications for platelet concentrate transfusions?

Prophylactic:
1. All patients with platelet counts less than 20,000
2. Before, during, or after surgery or invasive procedure with platelet count less than 50,000

Therapeutic:
1. Significant bleeding and platelet count less than 50,000
2. Significant bleeding in the setting of platelet dysfunction, no matter what the platelet count (e.g., mediastinal bleeding after cardiopulmonary bypass)

Volume of 1 unit of random donor platelet concentrate?

~ 50 ml

Number of random donor units in 1 unit of single donor platelet concentrate?

6–8

How much does 1 random donor unit raise the platelet count?

5000–10,000

What are some adverse effects of platelet transfusions?

1. Transfusion reactions (up to 30% have a nonhemolytic febrile reaction, the highest of any blood product)
2. Bacterial transmission (samples must be stored at room temperature). Remember: Cold platelets are dysfunctional.
3. Platelet-specific antibodies (platelets are the most immunogenic of all blood products). *The solution:* HLA-specific platelet concentrates.

What is heparin-induced thrombocytopenia?

An autoimmune destruction of platelets by cross-reacting antibodies (IgG) to heparin

What is the incidence of heparin-induced thrombocytopenia?

~ 5% of all patients on therapeutic doses of heparin

What are the clinical features of heparin-induced thrombocytopenia?

1. Thrombocytopenia (often less than 50,000) develops about 1 week after exposure to heparin of any dose via any route, including SQ injections or central line flushes, and may develop sooner if previously exposed to heparin.

2. 1% of patients with heparin-induced thrombocytopenia develop arterial and/or venous thrombi as part of the syndrome; life-threatening in 30%.
3. Excessive bleeding is a rare complication.

How is heparin-induced thrombocytopenia diagnosed?

Usually presumptive (in the appropriate clinical setting), as detection of heparin-platelet-antibody complexes in patient's serum has low sensitivity and specificity

What is the treatment for heparin-induced thrombocytopenia?

1. Discontinue all heparin (including catheter flushes and heparin locks).
2. Use alternative anticoagulation agents (if necessary): Coumadin, ancrod, low–molecular-weight dextran.
Note: Low–molecular-weight heparin, although less immunogenic, is not an acceptable substitute.

What is the prognosis for a patient diagnosed with heparin-induced thrombocytopenia?

Excellent, if diagnosed before onset of severe thrombocytopenia or thromboses. Therefore, the platelet count should be monitored daily in all patients after the institution of heparin therapy.

COAGULATION, ANTICOAGULATION, AND DISORDERS OF SECONDARY HEMOSTASIS

What is secondary hemostasis?

Formation of a cross-linked fibrin clot

Which clotting factors are unstable at temperatures above 4°C?

Factors V and VIII. Therefore, these factors are found at low levels in whole blood (stored at 4°C or higher); in fresh frozen plasma (stored at temperatures lower than 0°), they are present at adequate levels for therapeutic replacement of these factors.

Which is the only clotting factor not produced by the liver?

Factor VIII (made by endothelial cells)

Pathways of the coagulation cascade?

Extrinsic: (factor VII); intrinsic (factors XII, XI, IX, VIII); and common (factors X, V, XIII, thrombin, fibrinogen)

What does the PTT measure?	Activity of the intrinsic pathway
What prolongs the PTT?	Heparin, inherited factor deficiencies (e.g., hemophilia A and B), liver disease, DIC, severe vitamin K deficiency (common pathway), supratherapeutic warfarin doses (common pathway), von Willebrand syndrome, lupus anticoagulant
What is heparin?	A naturally occurring mucopolysaccharide polymer obtained from bovine and porcine sources for clinical use
How does heparin work?	Potentiates the effects of antithrombin III, which degrades several clotting factors (including thrombin)
How is heparin administered?	Parenterally: IV (systemic anticoagulation); SQ (DVT prophylaxis); intra-arterially (vascular surgery); catheter flushes (to maintain patency)
How are the effects of heparin monitored?	PTT or activated clotting time (ACT) [heparin elevates both at therapeutic doses]
What is the duration of action of heparin?	$T_{1/2}$ less than 1 hour. If the patient is on heparin drip, stop at least 4 hours before surgery or invasive procedure.
Can the effects of heparin be reversed/neutralized?	Yes, with IV protamine sulfate
What does the PT measure?	Activity of the extrinsic pathway
What is the INR?	A newer and more uniform means of monitoring warfarin therapy by eliminating the wide variability in PT measurements as a result of different lab techniques and reagents used

What prolongs the PT?
1. Warfarin
2. Vitamin K deficiency
3. Liver disease (decreased factor VII synthesis)
4. DIC
5. Supratherapeutic heparin doses (common pathway)

What are some causes of vitamin K deficiency?
1. Malnutrition
2. Malabsorption (interruption of enterohepatic circulation of bile acids, terminal ileal disease)
3. Broad-spectrum antibiotics (eradication of endogenous vitamin K–producing gut flora)
4. Normal neonate (no gut flora)

How does warfarin work?
Inhibits vitamin K reductase and thus the activity of the vitamin K–dependent factors (II, VII, IX, X, protein C, protein S)

Why is the PT prolonged before the PTT?
Factor VII (extrinsic pathway) has the shortest $T_{1/2}$ and is therefore inhibited at the lowest warfarin doses. At higher doses, the common pathway is inhibited, resulting in prolongation of both the PT and PTT.

What are the clinical uses of warfarin?
Long-term prophylactic (e.g., mechanical valves) or therapeutic (e.g., DVT) anticoagulation

How is warfarin administered?
Orally

How are the effects of warfarin reversed?
1. Immediately with fresh frozen plasma (Rule of thumb: 1 unit decreases the PT by 2 seconds)
2. Slowly (within 4 hours) with vitamin K (SQ, IM, or IV). (Vitamin K IV in small increments can quickly bring down PT.)

What is Virchow's triad?
1. Endothelial trauma
2. Stasis
3. Hypercoagulability
These three factors conspire to cause DVT.

What are common risk factors for DVT?	Age older than 40 years, cancer, obesity, major surgery (especially operations on the abdomen, pelvis, or lower extremities), varicose veins, congestive heart failure, myocardial infarction, stroke, soft tissue trauma and fractures of the leg, estrogen use, prolonged immobilization/paralysis, hypercoagulable states
What are hypercoagulable states?	Antithrombin III deficiency, protein C or S deficiency, resistance to activated protein C, dysfibrinogenemia, lupus anticoagulant, heparin-induced thrombocytopenia, polycythemia vera, hyperviscosity syndromes, thrombocytosis
Overall, what is the most common condition associated with DVT?	Pregnancy
What is the most significant complication of DVT?	PE
What are the long-term sequelae of DVT?	Postphlebitic syndrome (venous insufficiency, venous stasis ulcers), recurrent DVTs
Where do most DVTs begin?	Deep veins of the calf
What is the source of most PEs?	Iliac and femoral veins
What is the intent of DVT prophylaxis?	To prevent the potentially life-threatening sequelae of PE
What is adequate prophylaxis for a patient at low risk for thromboembolism?	Early ambulation and elastic stockings
Moderate risk?	Low-dose heparin (5000 units SQ, q12 hours) or intermittent pneumatic compression

High risk?

Low-dose heparin (5000 units SQ, q8 hours) or low–molecular-weight heparin (once daily)

Very high risk?

Low-dose or low–molecular-weight heparin *and* intermittent pneumatic compression or low-to-moderate warfarin anticoagulation (especially for hip fractures, hip surgery, other very high-risk orthopaedic procedures)

What is Homan's sign?

Pain on forced dorsiflexion of the foot. Suggests a DVT, but only present in $\frac{1}{3}$ of patients with a thrombus.

How are DVTs diagnosed?

1. Duplex ultrasonography—the initial procedure of choice. Better for proximal thrombi (iliac, femoral veins), unreliable for distal thrombi (calf veins). A negative study in a high-risk patient should be repeated in a few days to detect proximal extension of a distal thrombus or confirmed with venography.
2. Venography—the "gold standard." Reliably detects both proximal and distal thrombi. Its greatest utility is in confirming an equivocal or negative ultrasound exam in a patient considered to be at high risk for a DVT.
3. Impedance plethysmography (IPG)—as a result of its low sensitivity and specificity, this diagnostic modality has been virtually replaced by ultrasonography.

What is standard therapy for DVT?

Five days of IV heparin (PTT 1.5–2X normal), followed by at least 3 months of warfarin anticoagulation (INR 2–3). Current recommendation is for 6 months of anticoagulation.

What are indications for placement of a vena cava (Greenfield) filter?

1. Patient at high risk for thromboembolism in whom anticoagulation is contraindicated
2. PE while receiving adequate anticoagulation therapy

What is DIC?	Disseminated intravascular coagulation (DIC) is a systemic syndrome triggered by a variety of clinical situations and disease processes; it is characterized by both hemorrhage and intravascular thrombosis, often resulting in end-organ dysfunction.
Most significant cause of morbidity and mortality from DIC?	End-organ dysfunction from diffuse vascular thromboses. (*Not* hemorrhage, although this is often the most obvious manifestation!)

What conditions are associated with DIC?

1. Obstetric problems (amniotic fluid embolism, retained fetus, eclampsia, abortion, abruptio placentae)
2. Massive transfusion
3. Hemolytic transfusion reaction
4. Bacterial sepsis (gram-negative or gram-positive)
5. Viremia (HIV, cytomegalovirus, varicella-zoster virus, hepatitis)
6. Malignancy (metastatic solid tumors and leukemias)
7. Trauma (especially crush injuries associated with extensive soft tissue devitalization)
8. Liver disease
9. Cardiovascular disorders
10. Intravascular prostheses/devices (intra-aortic balloon pump, vascular grafts, peritoneovenous shunts)

What macromolecules can trigger DIC?	Thromboplastin, tissue factor, subendothelial collagen
Which two enzymes must *both* be active in the systemic circulation for DIC to develop?	Thrombin and plasmin
What are the effects of circulating thrombin?	Diffuse intravascular thromboses and end-organ damage
What are the effects of circulating plasmin?	Impaired hemostasis and diffuse hemorrhages

What are fibrin degradation products (FDPs)?

Breakdown products of plasmin's enzymatic action on fibrinogen and fibrin monomers

How are D-dimer fragments formed?

Plasmin-mediated cleavage of cross-linked fibrin

Common lab abnormalities in DIC?

1. Elevated PT and PTT (plasmin-mediated lysis of clotting factors, FDP interference with fibrin monomer polymerization)
2. Thrombocytopenia (platelet-trapping in diffuse microvascular fibrin clots)
3. Hypofibrinogenemia (plasmin-mediated)
4. Increased FDP titers
5. Increased D-dimer fragments (this is the most reliable test)
6. Increased bleeding time (FDP-mediated platelet dysfunction)
7. Decreased antithrombin levels

What is the treatment for low-grade DIC?

1. Treat underlying cause (often the only therapy necessary).
2. Antiplatelet agents (e.g., aspirin)
3. SQ heparin (if no response to above measures)

What is the treatment for fulminant DIC?

(Note: Some aspects remain controversial.)
1. Treat inciting disease process (sometimes all that is required).
2. Halt intravascular coagulation; low-dose SQ or IV heparin (equally effective), antiplatelet agents (aspirin), antithrombin concentrates.
3. If still bleeding after above measures, replace platelets (platelet concentrates) and clotting factors (FFP, cryoprecipitate) based on laboratory values.
4. Finally, consider inhibition of fibrinolysis (ϵ-aminocaproic acid or tranexamic acid) only if above measures have failed. These agents may precipitate fatal thromboses if patient is not anticoagulated first.

16

Skin, Musculoskeletal System

What are some health maintenance issues related to the skin of the patient in the ICU?

1. Frequently turn patient to avoid pressure sores.
2. Avoid sheet burn (cover areas that a moving patient may abrade).
3. Do NOT pad pressure points; pad AROUND pressure points. (Even a soft pad on a pressure point keeps the pressure on that point.)
4. Greasy skin is healthy skin (prescribe lotions, etc.).
5. Apply antifungal powder to moist areas such as groins.
6. Consider mechanized air bed for patient who will be immobile for a long time.
7. Make sure tubes (especially nasogastric tubes and Foleys) are not causing skin necrosis.
8. Minimize tape. Try to eliminate tape from chest. Do not use stretchy tapes.
9. Get iodine-containing compounds off skin ASAP.
10. Be sure skin's nutritional needs are met (intravenous fat, zinc supplementation, vitamin C, other vitamins).
11. Do not culture skin. This practice wastes time and money.
12. Order sheet cradles and sheep skin heel protection for patients with ischemic lower extremities.
13. Be sure heat lamps aren't too close, especially to ischemic skin.
14. Inspect all wounds daily, more often if patient is febrile.
15. Look at back side of patient by logrolling each day.

16. Always prescribe some form of physical therapy.
17. Minimize edema.

What type of suture material causes the least tissue inflammation over the long term when used to secure a central venous line or other apparatus to the skin?

Fine monofilament suture. Braided suture is inclined to produce and aggravate skin infections.

What is the normal core temperature in humans?

36°C–37.5°C

Describe the normal diurnal variation in core temperature.

There is a temperature nadir in the morning hours, and a temperature peak in the evening.

Name some methods used by the body to limit heat loss or gain.

Sweating, shivering, vasodilatation, and vasoconstriction

Name some methods used by the physician to limit heat loss or gain.

Heat lamps, warm IV fluids, blankets, warm respiratory gases in ventilators, sponge baths. More aggressive measures include gastric or colonic lavage with iced saline or cooling blankets.

Is fever dangerous to febrile patients?

Not unless it is causing cardiac compromise or unless the temperature gets above 40°C. (There may even be some survival advantage to being febrile, as shown in animal studies.)

Name some ways to avoid or treat dry skin in the ICU.

Keep bathing to a minimum, use extra-fatted soaps, and use emollients to keep skin lubricated.

Name some ways to treat pruritus.

Topical agents such as camphor, phenol compounds, or calamine lotions may be helpful. Systemic antihistamines are useful, especially for urticaria, which consists of raised, erythematous, pruritic plaques.

What is intertrigo?

Intertrigo is an eruption occurring in skinfold areas due to skin rubbing together. These areas may be colonized by yeast or bacteria. Treatment consists of keeping the skin in the affected area cool and dry, keeping the skin in the fold separated, and application of topical steroids.

What are decubitus ulcers?

Pressure sores resulting from skin necrosis due to continuous pressure in areas of bony prominence. (Remember that 'decubitus' is an adjective and not a noun.)

Most common areas for decubitus ulcers in ICU patients?

Sacrum, heels, hips, back of skull, lateral foot, knees, ankles

Patients at increased risk?

1. All who are bedridden or immobile (ventilated patients, debilitated patients, and patients with neurologic deficits, especially spinal cord injuries)
2. Patients who have ischemic areas (sacrum after aortobifemoral bypass or distal foot)
3. Those who have periods of low cardiac output

How may they be prevented?

Decubitus ulcers should virtually never happen. Frequent turning, good skin hygiene (keeping skin clean and dry), cushions, air flotation beds, and nutrition monitoring are effective preventive measures. Remember to avoid padding pressure points. Pad areas around pressure points.

What aspects of nursing care are particularly important in prevention?

1. Primary pressure relief (i.e., pillow between legs to avoid pressure ulcers at the knees and ankles)
2. Turning schedules: q1–2 hours in immobile patient; newer devices such as airflow mattresses may lessen necessity for turning.

Define a stage I pressure ulcer.

Pressure sore characterized by persistent nonbleeding erythema over a bony surface in contact with another bony surface or a continuous pressure source; characterized by an intact epidermis.

What is responsible for the persistent nonbleeding erythema in a stage I pressure ulcer?

Thrombosed microcirculation beneath the epidermis

Define a stage II pressure ulcer.

Similar to stage I ulcer but with partial-thickness skin loss involving epidermis or dermis or both; characterized by blister or shallow crater formation

Should these blisters be debrided?

This is a point of some controversy. However, most recently it is generally felt that if there is no sign of infection, there is no need to debride.

Define a stage III pressure ulcer.

Pressure sore characterized by the presence of ulcer formation without undermining of adjacent tissue, but extending through the epidermis and dermis into subcutaneous fat; does not extend to muscle, fascia, or bone.

Define a stage IV pressure ulcer.

Similar to stage III lesion, but the ulceration extends into muscle, fascia, bone, or supporting structures (i.e., tendon)

Which pressure ulcers should be debrided?

Debridement seems to be the best strategy in stage III and stage IV ulcers.

What function does debridement serve in care of the ulcer?

Serves to remove medium for bacterial growth from wound surface (i.e., nonviable tissue)

Are surface cultures of any value in this setting?

NO!

Do positive surface cultures warrant antibiotics?

No, unless other signs of sepsis are present

Why not?	Increased risk of creating resistant organisms, and you shouldn't treat surface colonization, only invasive infections.
Are deep biopsies helpful in the treatment of pressure ulcers?	Yes. These must be done for both qualitative and quantitative analysis.
What minimum concentration of invading organisms indicates a true wound infection?	100,000 organisms/g of tissue (10^5/g)
Will an infected wound/ ulcer heal without antibiotics?	No
What other signs/symptoms should alert the physician to a possible infected ulcer?	Fever, tachycardia, zone of erythema around the ulcer, purulent discharge from the ulcer
Can a patient with poor nutrition develop a pressure ulcer despite good nursing care?	No
An elderly diabetic patient has had one leg revascularized and is bedridden. He is lying recumbent for a week. What site on both lower extremities is subject to pressure ischemia and skin breakdown if not properly protected?	The heels are commonly the site of development of pressure sores in bedridden patients in the circumstance just described.
What are some skin manifestations associated with gastrointestinal bleeding?	Cutaneous signs of cirrhosis and portal hypertension (i.e., jaundice, spider angiomata, palmar erythema, caput medusa, alopecia, etc.)
What are the cutaneous signs which may be associated with thrombocytopenia?	Petechiae, purpura, ecchymoses

Name the cutaneous signs associated with hemorrhagic pancreatitis.

Grey-Turner's sign (flank ecchymosis) and Cullen's sign (periumbilical ecchymosis). These occur in 1% of cases and suggest severe hemorrhagic pancreatitis.

What is a cutaneous manifestation often associated with an acute abdomen?

Cutaneous hyperesthesia may be present in the patient with an acute abdomen and is associated with inflammation/irritation of the underlying parietal peritoneum.

What is Stevens-Johnson syndrome?

This is a severe form of erythema multiforme with marked oral mucosal and ocular involvement. It has a variable but usually less severe cutaneous component. These patients often develop extensive epidermal necrosis with large denuded areas.

How is the diagnosis made?

This syndrome is diagnosed clinically because the histologic picture may not be helpful, particularly in the early stages.

Are systemic corticosteroids useful in Stevens-Johnson syndrome?

The use of systemic corticosteroids in the treatment of Stevens-Johnson syndrome is controversial. They may be useful in symptomatic patients with rapidly evolving severe disease; however, cortocosteroid use may be associated with a higher complication rate and prolongation of disease.

What conditions most commonly account for the mortality in Stevens-Johnson syndrome?

Bacterial septicemia, fluid-electrolyte abnormalities, and organ failure. This condition is the equivalent of a large burn.

What patients are most at risk for disseminated varicella-zoster infection (with visceral involvement)?

This occurs in only about 2% of patients with "shingles" but in a much higher percentage of immunosuppressed patients with underlying Hodgkin's disease or other conditions.

What is the etiology of this disorder?

This occurs as a sequela to primary (varicella) or recurrent (herpes zoster) infections. The varicella-zoster virus can be responsible for life-threatening infections such as encephalitis and pneumonitis.

What is the usual presentation in the patient with disseminated varicella-zoster virus?

Cough, respiratory difficulty, chest pain, or neurologic abnormalities may be seen in a patient with an antecedent dermatomal herpes zoster or chickenpox. Viral pneumonitis and encephalitis are ominous clinical developments in these patients.

What is the dermatologic sign of dissemination in a patient with herpes zoster?

Multiple vesicular lesions occurring away from the original dermatome of involvement

How is disseminated varicella-zoster virus diagnosed?

Initially by the clinical picture and a positive Tzanck smear, confirmed by viral cultures

What is the usual management of such patients?

Acyclovir is the most effective preventive and therapeutic agent. Patients should be managed in an ICU setting once the diagnosis of dissemination with internal organ involvement is known.

What percentage of all medical inpatients are affected by skin eruptions?

About 2%–3%

What conditions are included in this class of skin disorders?

Morbilliform, urticarial, and bullous eruptions as well as erythema multiforme, Stevens-Johnson syndrome, and toxic epidermal necrolysis

Which medications are most commonly associated with the development of morbilliform skin eruptions?

The greatest incidence occurs with the penicillins, sulfonamides, phenytoin, and barbiturates. Blood products also produce a high incidence of eruptions.

Describe the typical eruption.

It is usually erythematous and maculopapular and initially occurs on the trunk or in dependent areas. The macules and papules are usually symmetric and tend to become confluent.

When associated with medications, how long before the rash appears?

The typical eruption occurs within the first 7 days of initiation of therapy, but may take as long as 28 days to appear (ampicillin).

How are such conditions treated?

If feasible, the offending agent should be discontinued. Pruritis is treated with topical antipruritics such as hydrocortisone cream or Sarna lotion. Oral antihistamines are used to relieve the itching. The key to cutaneous therapy is evaporation, using periodic open wet dressings followed by a mild steroid ointment, either hydrocortisone or a nonfluorinated steroid.

Is anaphylaxis likely if an agent that causes a skin eruption is continued?

Probably not. A drug may be continued in the face of a morbilliform eruption with little fear of an anaphylactic episode.

Urticarial eruptions are secondary to what?

Many urticarial eruptions, especially acute urticaria, are secondary to a medication. Other causes of urticarial eruptions include neoplasia, collagen vascular disease, infections, and other chronic diseases.

What is the usual time course of these reactions?

Such eruptions may occur within minutes of administration of the drug as an anaphylactic reaction, within 12 to 36 hours as part of an IgE-dependent accelerated reaction, or up to 7 to 10 days as a serum sickness syndrome.

What is the clinical appearance of this reaction?

The dermis is infiltrated with fluid, giving an indurated orange-peel appearance to the skin. The lesions may be quite large and dependent areas may be accompanied by purpura. The plaques resolve within 12 to 24 hours without residuals.

How is an urticarial eruption managed?	Identify and discontinue the offending medication. Oral antihistamines of the H_1 type are the mainstay of therapy. Severe cases associated with wheezing, laryngeal edema, and circulatory collapse may require subcutaneous epinephrine, tracheal intubation, and systemic steroids.
Name some causes of bullous drug reactions.	Drug alone, drug plus light, and drug overdoses ("coma blisters"). Specific etiologies include bromides, iodides, mercury, arsenic, salicylates, phenolphthalein, minoxidil, and penicillamine.
How are typical bullous drug reactions managed?	Therapy consists of discontinuing the causative agent and using supportive skin care. Large bullae may require aspiration and topical antibiotics.
What medications are known to cause phototoxic bullous drug reactions?	Furosemide, tetracycline, psoralen, and nalidixic acid
What is purpura?	Purpura is a condition characterized by diffuse hemorrhage into the skin.
What are petechiae?	Petechiae are hemorrhagic macules less than 3 mm in diameter.
What are ecchymoses?	Ecchymoses are hemorrhagic macules greater than 3 mm in diameter.
What causes contact dermatitis?	It can be due to an allergy or an irritant, with the latter being the most common.
What does "classic" contact dermatitis look like?	Vesicles on an erythematous base, in a linear arrangement, are the hallmarks of this condition.
Is this pattern a generalized finding on the patient?	Typically the eruption is localized to the area of the contact.

How is a contact dermatitis generally treated?

Discontinue the topical medication or irritant. Apply open wet dressings followed by a topical steroid ointment. Antihistamines may be useful, and oral steroids are indicated in an acute contact dermatitis that is widespread.

What are the primary musculoskeletal concerns of the critically ill patient?

1. Keep muscles moving, even if passively.
2. Avoid contractures, even if splints are required.
3. Stabilize broken bones, even if only with air splints.

How much blood can a patient lose from a pelvic fracture?

Their entire blood volume

What strategies can be used if a pelvic fracture continues to bleed?

1. Military antishock trouser compression
2. Angiography with embolization
3. Operative fixation

What is a compartment syndrome?

Increased pressure in a closed space causing direct injury and impairing blood flow through the area

Where in the body are compartment syndromes most common?

Forearm and calf

Under what conditions should you be more vigilant in looking for compartment syndromes?

After periods of ischemia (after revascularization or removal of intra-aortic balloon pump), after trauma (fractures, crush injuries, electrical injuries)

What are some examples of "nontraditional" compartment syndromes?

1. Increased intracranial pressure
2. Tension pneumothorax
3. Cardiac tamponade
4. Increased intra-abdominal pressure

What bones should be x-rayed in the secondary or even tertiary surveys in trauma patients?

1. Every bone that has a skin abnormality over it
2. Any area that is tender or swollen

What is fat embolism syndrome?

A constellation of signs and symptoms that occurs after major bone injury, in which the lungs are showered with fat released from the bone marrow; can result in adult respiratory distress syndrome or DIC in most severe cases

What is the "classic" triad for diagnosis of fat embolism syndrome?

1. Hypoxia
2. Confusion
3. Petechiae over the upper body

What is rhabdomyolysis?

Acute destruction of skeletal muscle

What can cause rhabdomyolysis?

Crush injuries, electrical burns, acute muscular ischemia, seizures, infections, hypokalemia, toxins, and hypophosphatemia (among others)

How is rhabdomyolysis dangerous to the patient's overall health?

The resultant myoglobinuria can lead to acute tubular necrosis (ATN) and renal failure. Also, electrolyte and acid–base disturbances secondary to washout of injured muscle (lactic acid, K^+, etc.) can cause cardiac embarrassment.

How can one diagnose rhabdomyolysis?

1. Urinalysis positive for blood
2. No urinary erythrocytes
3. Urinary myoglobin assay

What is the treatment for rhabdomyolysis?

Stop underlying muscle destruction. Also, attempts can be made to prevent ATN by producing a brisk, alkaline diuresis with fluids, mannitol, and bicarbonate. In extreme cases, consideration may be given to early amputation to protect the patient's life. Also, one must treat acidosis and hyperkalemia aggressively.

Section 3

Pathologic Processes in the ICU

17   Malnutrition

What are the indications for nutritional support?

1. The progressive loss of 10% of a patient's ideal body weight during a 4–6 month period
2. Ideal body weight less than 90%
3. A rapid weight loss of more than 6% of body weight may mean a direct loss of muscle protein, which may be insufficient to maintain caloric needs.
4. Objectively: a serum albumin of less than 3.0 g/dl. (sAlb, a protein manufactured in the liver, is an indicator of long-term nutritional status. Serum pre-albumin is also a liver product, but has a shorter half-life, on the order of 1 day, and is an indicator of short-term nutrition and thus replenishment.

What are the human body's basal caloric needs?

1. 25–35 kcal/kg/24 hours unless stressed. But remember, carbohydrates produce CO_2, which must be removed from the body by ventilation; as most ICU patients are being mechanically ventilated, increased CO_2 production delays weaning;
2. 1.0–1.5 g of protein/kg/24 hours. Remember, protein metabolism generates nitrogenous waste as N_2, which is excreted by the kidneys and must be modified for patients with renal disease. There is 1 g of N_2 in 6.25 g of protein.

What is the golden rule of surgical nutritional support?

If the gut works, use it.

ENTERAL NUTRITION

When is supplemental enteral nutrition considered routine care?

1. Protein-calorie malnutrition, with inadequate oral intake of nutrients over the previous 5 days
2. Normal nutritional status but less than half of required oral intake of nutrients for the previous 7–10 days
3. Severe dysphagia
4. Major full-thickness burns
5. Massive small bowel resection in combination with administration of total parenteral nutrition (TPN)
6. Low-output enterocutaneous fistulas

When is supplemental enteral nutrition usually helpful?

1. Major trauma
2. Radiation therapy
3. Mild chemotherapy
4. Liver failure and severe renal dysfunction

When is enteral nutrition of limited or undetermined value?

1. Intensive chemotherapy
2. Immediate postoperative period or poststress period
3. Acute enteritis
4. More than 90% resection of small bowel

When is enteral nutrition contraindicated?

1. Complete, mechanical intestinal obstruction
2. Ileus or intestinal hypomotility
3. Severe diarrhea
4. High-output external fistulas
5. Severe, acute pancreatitis
6. Shock
7. Aggressive nutritional support not desired by the patient or legal guardian
8. Prognosis not warranting aggressive nutritional support

What are some complications of enteral nutrition?

1. Aspiration. This complication can kill your patients. Be careful!
2. Diarrhea
3. Metabolic abnormalities (hyperkalemia, hypokalemia, hyponatremia, hyperglycemia, hypophosphatemia)

What is the preferred route of nutritional support in the ICU?	"If the gut works, use it." Enteral feedings are cheaper, equally effective, and pose fewer complications. Also, they reduce villous atrophy and bacterial translocation.
What is the top priority in enteral nutrition?	To be as certain as you possibly can to keep the food in the gut, preferably beyond the pylorus. The lungs are a very poor place to absorb nutrients!
What is the major risk when initiating enteral feedings in an ICU patient?	Aspiration and subsequent aspiration pneumonitis
What conditions place the ICU patient at high risk for aspiration?	Endotracheal intubation, sedation or obtundation, nasogastric intubation, H_2-blockers, and supine positioning. Remember—a tube in the airway does not prevent aspiration. Patients aspirate around cuffs.
What can be done to reduce the incidence of aspiration in patients receiving enteral nutrition?	Transpyloric or jejunal feedings. When using the gastric route, elevate head to $45°$, discontinue H_2-blockers, and stop if gastric residuals are over 150 ml or if gastric dilation seems to be present by examination or chest x-ray.
What is the most frequent complication seen in patients receiving enteral nutrition?	Diarrhea. This can be treated by changing rate or osmolality. Opiates useful after infectious etiologies excluded.

TOTAL PARENTERAL NUTRITION

What is the maximum dextrose concentration allowable for peripheral parenteral nutrition?	10% dextrose. Greater concentrations will sclerose peripheral veins and therefore require central venous access.
What components can be ordered in TPN solution?	Dextrose, amino acids, lipids, electrolytes, vitamins, minerals, trace elements, and/or insulin, heparin, and H_2-blockers.

What change in TPN can be made for a ventilator-dependent patient with a respiratory quotient (RQ) > 1.0?

Reduce the carbohydrate-to-lipid ratio to lower CO_2 production and ease the respiratory burden of CO_2 clearance; i.e., use more lipids.

What laboratory studies are used to monitor ICU patients receiving TPN?

Daily electrolytes, BUN, and creatinine; blood glucose; SMA-12 and magnesium daily for 3 days, and twice weekly thereafter.

How do branched chain amino acids (BCAA) benefit patients with hepatic failure/ dysfunction?

BCAAs (valine, leucine, isoleucine) are metabolized by skeletal muscle and thereby avoid hepatic processing for energy production. They also lessen encephalopathy by decreasing aromatic amino acid transport across the blood–brain barrier.

What are the considerations when writing TPN orders for patients with renal failure?

Appropriate fluid and electrolyte restrictions. Low protein input to minimize azotemia. Adequate provision of carbohydrate calories to maintain nitrogen balance in face of low protein input.

When is TPN considered routine care?

1. Malabsorption
- Massive small bowel resection
- Impaired intestinal motility and absorption associated with small bowel diseases
- Radiation enteritis
- Protracted diarrhea
2. Bone marrow transplant patients receiving high-dose chemotherapy or radiation
3. Moderate to severe pancreatitis
4. Patients who have lost more than 10% of usual body weight
5. Catabolic patients with or without evidence of malnutrition when GI tract cannot be used for 5–7 days

When is TPN usually helpful?

1. After major surgery when an adequate enteral diet will not be resumed within 7–10 days
2. After stresses such as moderate trauma or burns of 30%–50% of body

surface area, when an enteral diet cannot be resumed for more than 7–10 days

3. Enterocutaneous fistula
4. Inflammatory bowel disease
5. Hyperemesis gravidarum
6. In patients for whom adequate enteral nutrition cannot be initiated within 7–10 days of hospitalization
7. Small bowel obstruction secondary to inflammatory lesions
8. Preoperatively (over 7–10 days)

When is TPN of limited value?

1. Functional GI tract within a 10-day period in a well-nourished patient who endures minimal stress or trauma
2. Untreatable disease
3. Immediate postoperative period

When is TPN contraindicated?

1. In a patient with a functional and usable GI tract
2. During a period of nutritional support estimated to be fewer than 5 days
3. When the risks of TPN are believed to exceed the potential benefits

COMPLICATIONS OF TOTAL PARENTERAL NUTRITION?

Complications	Possible Causes
Hematologic	Deficiencies of iron, vitamin B_{12}, copper, or folic acid
Gastrointestinal	
Gallstone sludge	Prolonged (4–6 wk) continuous parenteral nutrition
Increased liver function tests (LFTs)	Overfeeding (fatty liver)
Pancreatitis	Hypertriglyceridemia, hypercalcemia
Mechanical	
Air embolism	Air enters open needle or catheter during insertion
Catheter embolism	Venous catheter sheared as pulled through introducer needle
Catheter misplacement	Subclavian catheter into ipsilateral jugular vein, etc.
Pneumothorax	Insertion needle penetrates apical pleura
Thoracic duct laceration	Attempt to catheterize left subclavian vein

Complications of Total Parenteral Nutrition? (continued)

Complications	Possible Causes
Venous thrombosis	Location of catheter (femoral vein), prolonged use of vein
Metabolic	
Azotemia	Renal insufficiency, too much protein
Hyperchloremia metabolic acidosis	Excess chloride content of crystalline amino acids
Hypocalcemia	Inadequate administration; hypoalbuminemia; after phosphorus repletion without calcium
Altered coagulation	Hypertriglyceridemia
Cyanosis	Altered pulmonary diffusion capacity
Essential fatty acid (FA) deficiency	Lack of essential FA (linoleic acid, linolenic acid) in TPN
Pyrogenic reaction	Secondary to Intralipid
Hypertriglyceridemia	Rapid fat infusion; decreased clearance
Hyperglycemia (glycosuria, osmotic diuresis, ketoacidosis, hyperosmolar nonketonic coma)	Inadequate endogenous or exogenous insulin; excess dose or rate of infusion of dextrose
Hypoglycemia	Persistence of exogenous insulin production 2° to prolonged stimulation of islet cells of high carbohydrate loads when TPN stopped
Hypomagnesemia	Inadequate administration; cisplatin
Hypermagnesemia	Excess administration; renal failure; antacids or laxatives
Osteomalacia	Excess aluminum in casein hydrolysates
Hypophosphatemia	Inadequate administration, especially when patient becomes anabolic after starvation (refeeding syndrome); diabetic ketoacidosis; intracellular shift 2° to excess dextrose
Hypokalemia	Diuresis; inadequate intake; increased protein anabolism (refeeding)
Hyperkalemia	Excess administration; renal failure; metabolic acidosis
Night blindness	Deficiency of vitamin A (long-term TPN; Crohn's disease)
Refeeding syndrome	Aggressive TPN in malnourished patient; excess carbohydrate and sodium, hypophosphatemia
Sepsis	
Candidemia	Phagocyte dysfunction in patient with hypophosphatemia; overgrowth of *Candida* in gut
Culture of catheter tip yields > 1000 organisms	Most common organisms are *Staphylococcus epidermidis, S. aureus, Klebsiella pneumonia, Candida albicans*

Where does nutritional support lie among patient care priorities in the ICU?

Airway, breathing, circulation, tissue oxygenation, acid–base balance, electrolyte balance, nutritional support

What are some relative indications for nutritional support in ICU patients?

1. Pre-existing malnutrition
2. When nutrition is not received for 5–7 days
3. An illness with expected course of 7–10 days or longer
4. Hypermetabolic conditions (sepsis, burns, pancreatitis)

When should an ICU patient undergo a nutritional status assessment?

On ICU day 2 and every 4–5 days thereafter

Which patients are at highest risk for malnutrition?

Those with pre-existing health problems, poor socioeconomic conditions, and severe injury or illness

What are some characteristics of protein malnutrition?

Poor wound healing, anergy, and decreased transferrin, albumin, prealbumin, lymphocytes. Hair is easily pluckable. Warning: The patient may look well nourished and still have protein malnutrition.

What is the Harris-Benedict equation and how is it used?

The equation used to determine basal metabolic rate (BMR) based on height, weight, age, and gender. Conversion factors are used for metabolic stressors (e.g., sepsis = $1.3 \times$ BMR).

What is the Fick method for determining caloric needs?

Indirect calorimetry via PA catheter that calculates oxygen consumption and converts to kcal per day

What is the metabolic profile and what information does it provide?

Indirect calorimetry via alveolar gas analysis to determine caloric needs and a respiratory quotient

What is the respiratory quotient (RQ) and how is it used?

RQ is the ratio of CO_2 production to O_2 consumption. Provides insight into substrate utilization: RQ = 1.0 with carbohydrate use; RQ = 0.7 with lipid use.

What are the protein requirements of a critically ill patient?

1.5–2.0 g/kg/day. This requirement is double that of unstressed patients and is necessary to counteract protein catabolism. Protein calories are not counted in calculating caloric needs.

Which tissues preferentially use glucose as an energy substrate?

Brain, red blood cells, and renal medulla use glucose exclusively when it is available.

How does the body store carbohydrates?

300 g glycogen are stored in liver and skeletal muscle and are converted to glucose by glucagon. This amount provides about 1,200 kcal in unfed state, which lasts about 24 hours.

What is the nitrogen balance?

Nitrogen balance describes metabolic status with respect to protein turnover. Positive balance indicates anabolism; negative balance indicates catabolism.

At what rate should carbohydrates be administered?

1 kcal/kg/hr will maintain nitrogen balance. Lesser rates lead to glycogenolysis and gluconeogenesis, whereas greater rates lead to lipogenesis (all of which expend energy).

What is "insulin resistance" and when does it occur?

Hyperglycemia despite elevated insulin levels; often seen in sepsis and severe trauma

Lipids should provide what portion of a patient's nonprotein calories (NPC)?

About 30% to provide a carbohydrate-to-lipid calorie ratio of 70:30, unless the patient is in respiratory failure, in which case lipid percentage should be higher

Excessive infusion of omega-6 lipid solutions (linoleic acid/soybean oil) can lead to what clinical problem?

Omega-6 fatty acid (FA) causes an increase in PGE_2 levels, which suppresses monocyte function. Use of omega-3 FA solutions does not increase PGE_2 levels and produces fewer immune-related complications.

18

Infection

What health maintenance issues related to infectious disease should be addressed frequently in your patients?

1. Obtain surveillance cultures occasionally (lines, sputum).
2. Check cultures, white blood cell count, differential.
3. Review antibiotics daily (trying to reduce number and duration).
4. Consider antifungal prophylaxis (nystatin powder, solutions, suppositories).
5. Consider antifungal treatment (unexplained sepsis, re-explorations, transplant patients).
6. Check all lines daily.

What are the five Ws of postoperative fever?

Wind (atelectasis, aspiration, pneumonia)
Water (urinary tract infection)
Wound (look at wound every day starting with postoperative day 1)
Walking (deep vein thrombosis [DVT], pulmonary edema [PE])
Wonder drug (drug allergies)

What is the standard work-up for fever in the ICU?

1. Blood cultures (including fungal if the patient has risk factors)
2. Sputum culture
3. Urine culture
4. Chest x-ray
5. Change or rewire central line if not done in the previous 72 hours.
6. Change arterial line. (Arterial lines are virtually never the source of infection in ICU patients and should be changed only if pus is evident at the site.)

What are the risk factors for infection in the ICU?

1. Immunocompromised patient
2. Multisystem organ failure (MSOF)
3. Total parenteral nutrition (TPN)
4. Broad spectrum antibiotic usage
5. Diabetes

What relatively unusual sites of infection are more prevalent in the ICU?

Central lines, sinuses, CNS

Why are sinuses at risk?

Because of tubes such as nasogastric (NG) tubes. The worst offenders are nasotracheal tubes.

What three etiologies account for persistent fever in the ICU?

1. Undiagnosed site of infection: lines, sinuses, CNS, abdomen, etc.
2. Noninfectious etiology: drugs
3. Organisms not treated by current antibiotics: resistant bacteria, viruses, and fungi. (If a patient remains persistently febrile in the ICU, especially a diabetic with a central line and receiving TPN, assume fungus until proven otherwise.)

What is SIRS?

Systemic inflammatory response syndrome, a term for the generalized immune response to illness; a.k.a. "sepsis." May or may not be due to infection.

What hemodynamic changes are associated with severe infection or sepsis?

Tachycardia, hypotension, increased cardiac output, decreased peripheral vascular resistance (PVR)

Which two cytokines most closely reproduce the septic response in animal models?

Interleukin-1, tumor necrosis factor

Which cytokine is most consistently elevated in clinical sepsis and is correlated with a bad outcome?

Interleukin-6

What is MSOF?

Multisystem organ failure or MODS, multiple organ dysfunction syndrome. MSOF is a condition associated in some cases with the end stage of sepsis and other systemic inflammatory syndromes.

What organ systems are most commonly affected by MODS?	1. Respiratory—respiratory insufficiency with difficulty with oxygenation and ventilation 2. Cardiovascular—hypotension shock 3. Renal—oliguria, anuria 4. Hepatic—hepatic liver enzyme dysfunction, hepatic synthetic function 5. Immune—untreatable sepsis
What are the approximate mortality rates associated with increasing numbers of systems involved?	1. One system = 10% 2. Two systems = 30% 3. Three systems = 70% 4. Four systems = 90% 5. Five systems = 100%
What is bacterial translocation?	The movement of enteric bacteria into normally sterile body spaces (e.g., lymph nodes, portal vein) despite an intact GI tract
What conditions are felt to predispose to translocation?	Severe trauma, burns, sepsis, absence of food in gut
Which bacteria most commonly translocate?	Gram-negative rods
What is the clinical relevance of translocation?	Unknown, but may predispose to the hematogenous spread of infection
Which fungus is most commonly isolated in the ICU?	*Candida albicans*
What conditions are felt to predispose to fungal infection?	Long-term antibacterial use, diabetes, fistulae, central venous catheters, severe illness, immunosuppression
What is the most common indication for the treatment of fungus in the ICU?	Multiple (more than three) sites of colonization, persistent fever, or leukocytosis despite adequate antibacterial coverage
What is the rationale for treating multiple sites of fungal colonization?	Retrospective studies have shown an association between more than three sites of colonization and eventual fungemia.

What are the common sites of colonization?

Urine, sputum, wound, nasopharynx, intertriginous folds

From simplest to most aggressive, what are the options for treating candiduria?

1. Remove Foley and reculture in 48 hours.
2. Intracystic instillation of amphotericin B for 3–5 days
3. IV fluconazole
4. IV amphotericin B

What is the usual dose of amphotericin B used to treat fungal infections in the ICU?

5–8 mg/kg total, as 0.3–0.5 mg/kg/day

How is amphotericin usually administered?

In a daily dose

What are the side effects of the administration of amphotericin?

The usual side effects are fever, rigors, vasodilatation.

How can these side effects be avoided?

Administration of amphotericin as a continuous infusion

What is the main side effect of continuously infused amphotericin?

Transient renal tubular dysfunction (increased creatinine, decreased potassium)

How can the sites of fungal growth be handled to attempt to decrease fungal infections?

1. Nystatin mouth rinse
2. Nystatin in gut
3. Mycostatin powder for intertriginous folds
4. Nystatin suppositories in vagina and rectum

When should amphotericin be given empirically?

1. For persistent fever or sepsis in an ICU patient thought to be covered with antibiotics
2. Re-explorations of immunocompromised patients
3. Bowel perforation

What two organisms require two-drug antibiotic therapy?

1. *Pseudomonas*
2. Enterococcus

What are the classic criteria for the diagnosis of nosocomial pneumonia?	Single or predominant organism on sputum culture with few squamous epithelial cells and many polys on gram stain, leukocytosis, pyrexia or hypothermia, new infiltrate on chest x-ray
What is the approximate mortality rate of nosocomial pneumonias in non-immunocompromised ventilated patients?	20%–40%
What is the importance of *Pseudomonas aeruginosa?*	Most common cause of nosocomial pneumonia
Which antibiotics have significant antipseudomonal activity?	Aminoglycosides, ceftazidime, aztreonam, antipseudomonal penicillins (piperacillin, mezlocillin, etc.) imipenem, ciprofloxacin
What is the treatment for significant *Enterococcus faecalis* infections?	High-dose ampicillin (or vancomycin) plus gentamicin
What is the treatment for significant *Enterobacter cloacae* or *Enterobacter aerogenes* infections?	An aminoglycoside (never a third-generation cephalosporin, due to the rapid development of resistance)
What central venous line locations have the greatest incidence of infection?	Femoral, internal jugular (IJ), with femoral having a higher incidence of infection than IJ
What central venous line locations have the least incidence of infection?	Subclavian
If a line is suspected of being infected, what do you do?	Rewire, culture
What culture result requires another line change?	More than 15 colonies of bacteria
What issues increase line infections?	TPN, high concentration dextrose solution, manipulations, difficult sites for dressings

What issues decrease line infections?	1. Changing lines over wires every 2–5 days 2. Keeping excellent dressings in place 3. Clean sites
A differential diagnosis of fever by organ systems can be made. What is the most common cause of fever in each of the following? 1. **CNS** 2. **Respiratory system** 3. **Cardiovascular system** 4. **GI system** 5. **Gastrourinary system** 6. **Hematologic system** 7. **Wounds** 8. **Skin** 9. **Monitoring equipment**	 1. Meningitis 2. Pneumonia, PE 3. Endocarditis 4. Gallbladder, colitis 5. Urinary tract infection 6. Transfusion reaction 7. Wound infection 8. Decubitus ulcers 9. Lines
Why are doctors and nurses so frequently vectors of disease in ICUs?	1. They don't wash their hands often enough. 2. They overprescribe antibiotics. 3. They don't pay enough attention to sterile technique.
What constitutes appropriate sterile technique for a procedure in the ICU?	1. Defat the skin. 2. Prep thoroughly with antiseptic solution. 3. Prep an area many, many times larger than seems necessary. 4. Use towels to block off site. 5. Cover everything with 3–4 feet of sterile drapes if possible. 6. Learn to gown and glove yourself (otherwise your cuffs are dirty). 7. Wear a mask. 8. Don't let the back end of J wires hit dirty objects. 9. Think like a germ!!!
What should be considered in a patient with fever and diarrhea, and/or leukocytosis?	Primarily *Clostridium difficile*
What is the treatment for C. difficile?	1. IV Flagyl or oral vancomycin 2. Stop antibiotics. 3. Recolonize bowel. 4. Get food in the gut.

19   Immunosuppression

What are some health maintenance issues for patients who are known to be immunosuppressed?

1. Follow blood counts to watch for marrow suppression.
2. Follow cyclosporine levels.
3. Monitor blood pressure and creatinine in a patient receiving cyclosporine.
4. Review prophylactic medications such as Bactrim and acyclovir to be sure they are being administered properly.
5. Pay extra attention to potential sites of occult infection (perineum, CNS, etc.).
6. Possible exposure to pathogens such as from contaminated water or exposure to people with communicable diseases

What types of patients are very immunosuppressed?

1. Transplant patients
2. Patients with AIDS

What types of patients are relatively immunosuppressed?

1. Patients with autoimmune diseases treated with immunosuppressive agents (arthritics treated with methotrexate)
2. Patients taking steroids (lung disease)
3. Severely injured patients (trauma, burns)

What types of patients are somewhat immunosuppressed?

1. Patients with diabetes
2. Patients who have just been on cardiopulmonary bypass
3. Patients at the extremes of age

Why is it important to have an idea of a patient's immune competency?

1. They may have infections or tumors that are difficult to find.
2. They may have unusual infections with organisms of low intrinsic pathogenicity, and they may have rapidly growing tumors.
3. They may have difficult-to-treat (resistant) infections or tumors.

What type of tumors do immunosuppressed patients have?

1. Transplant patients can have explosive or resistant growth of any type of tumor, but the most common tumor associated with immunosuppression is lymphoma. Other tumors are usually epithelial (skin, cervix, etc.).
2. AIDS patients can also have many tumors, but Kaposi's sarcoma is the classic AIDS-related tumor.

What type of infections can immunocompromised patients (including those on therapeutic steroids) have?

1. Any type of and even usually benign agents can be virulent.
2. Viral infections are common, especially the DNA viruses: cytomegalovirus, herpes simplex virus.
3. Also prone to contract *Pneumocystis carinii,* resistant tuberculosis, toxoplasmosis
4. Fungal infections are also prevalent.

What sort of work-up should you do for immunocompromised patients (including those on therapeutic steroids) who may have an infection?

1. Get a good history (exposures, animals in house, symptoms, prophylactic drugs being taken, history of the current illness, etc.).
2. Examine the patient. (Realize the abdominal examination will be less reliable than in the usual patient.)
3. Round up the usual suspects (blood, urine, sputum, chest x-ray).
4. Consider moving quickly to less common tests (lumbar puncture, chest and abdominal CT scan, sinus films, stool culture) guided by the clinical situation.
5. Remember that a patient taking steroids may have a normal abdominal examination, even in the situation of a perforated viscus; thus, you will want to get plain films of the abdomen, including an upright film to look for free air.

20 Neoplasia

What conditions are likely to end a cancer patient's life suddenly or prematurely?

1. Pulmonary embolism (PE)
2. Blood loss (e.g., hemoptysis from lung cancer)
3. Pericardial tamponade from malignant pleural effusion

What happens to the serum albumin in the typical cancer patient?

Albumin may be decreased from malignancy, chronic disease, or the presence of abnormal binding proteins (as seen in multiple myeloma).

In what two forms is calcium normally present in the serum?

About 1/2 exists as an ionized, free fraction and about 1/2 exists as a protein-bound fraction.

Name the plasma protein primarily involved in calcium transport.

Albumin

Which is the clinically relevant fraction that correlates best with signs and symptoms of hypercalcemia?

The unbound, ionized fraction

How do albumin levels relate to the ionized calcium level and thus hypercalcemia?

With decreases in serum albumin, the ionized fraction of calcium assumes a larger proportion of the total serum calcium, and total calcium levels may understate the severity of hypercalcemia.

Name a formula that relates changes in serum albumin to that of calcium.

In general, for every 1 g/dl decrease in the serum albumin, there is a 0.8 mg/dl decrease in the serum calcium.

What is a normal calcium level?

8–10 mg/dl

What is a normal ionized calcium level?

4.5 mg/dl

What serum level of calcium warrants urgent treatment?

Serum calcium levels more than 13 mg/dl, when corrected for changes in plasma proteins, or a clinical picture consistent with hypercalcemia, regardless of the serum calcium level, warrant urgent intervention.

What are the two most common causes of hypercalcemia?

1. Hyperparathyroidism
2. Malignancy

What is the mechanism of malignancy-associated hypercalcemia?

The most common cause is tumor production of a parathyroid hormone (PTH)-like (not PTH itself) peptide resulting in bone resorption. Less common causes are generation of osteoclast activating factor (OAF) or the production of other bone mobilizing peptides such as interleukin-1 and tumor necrosis factor (TNF) by tumors.

Hyperparathyroidism and malignancy account for what percentage of the total cases of hypercalcemia?

About 90% of the total

Solid tumors account for what percentage of cases of malignancy-associated hypercalcemia?

Solid tumors, particularly lung and breast carcinoma, account for about 80% of the total cases.

What are some other causes of hypercalcemia?

Other causes include vitamin D and vitamin A intoxication, sarcoidosis, immobility, milk alkali syndrome, renal failure, thyrotoxicosis, adrenal insufficiency, and medications such as thiazide, lithium, estrogens, and tamoxifen.

Hypercalcemia develops in what percentage of patients with malignancy?

10%–20%

What are the signs and symptoms of hypercalcemia?

1. Neuromuscular: muscle fatigue, weakness, psychosis, confusion, coma
2. Cardiovascular: hypertension, shortened QT interval, prolonged PR interval

3. GI: nausea, vomiting, and abdominal pain

Describe the patient in full-blown hypercalcemic crisis.

Such a patient may present with somnolence, lethargy, general weakness, abdominal pain, dehydration, renal failure, and nausea and vomiting.

How does hypercalcemia affect renal function?

Elevated serum calcium impairs the kidney's ability to concentrate urine, resulting in polyuria and polydipsia. An ensuing contraction alkalosis with dehydration leads to further renal impairment, and frank renal failure.

How is hypercalcemia treated acutely?

Levels greater than 13 mg/dl require prompt treatment, including hydration with normal saline to restore intravascular volume, followed by diuresis (furosemide) that enhances calciuresis by facilitating a provoked natriuresis.

What parenteral medications are effective in treating acute hypercalcemia?

Plicamycin, calcitonin, gallium nitrate, and hydroxyethane biphosphonate

Are cancer patients at increased risk for developing a PE?

Yes, they have a 2–3 times increased risk.

Name some causes of PE in the cancer patient.

1. Hypercoagulable state induced by the neoplasm or chemotherapy
2. Compression of vessels or obstruction of venous blood flow by tumor
3. Surgery (immobility, hypercoagulable state, etc.)

Can PE be a cause of sudden death?

Yes! It is one of only three causes of nontraumatic sudden death (the other two are ventricular fibrillation and aortic dissection).

PEs that result in sudden death usually occlude more than what percentage of the pulmonary vascular bed?

50%

Describe how a massive PE may result in sudden death.

The embolism causes a sudden reduction in the cross-sectional area of the pulmonary vascular bed. Cardiac output then falls, followed by hypoperfusion, shock, and death.

Why are prompt recognition and treatment so important in the patient suspected of having a PE?

75%–90% of those who die do so within the first few hours of the embolic event.

What is the overall mortality rate of PE?

If unrecognized and untreated, 30%

Where do most PEs originate?

In the deep venous system of the proximal lower extremities and, less commonly, in the pelvis

With what are clinically significant thrombi in the upper extremities and superior vena cava typically associated?

Indwelling catheters

What are the "classic" ECG findings in a patient with a PE?

The classic S1-Q3 pattern with right axis deviation and right bundle branch block. The ECG may actually be normal but often shows sinus tachycardia, inverted T waves or nonspecific ST-T wave abnormalities.

What should be the initial diagnostic test in a patient suspected of having a PE?

A radionuclide ventilation/perfusion (V/Q) scan

Does a normal V/Q scan rule out a PE?

A normal scan suggests less than a 1% chance of a major embolus.

What is the chance of an embolus with a high probability scan?

A high probability scan suggests more than an 85% chance of an embolus.

What is considered the "gold standard" in diagnosing a PE?

Pulmonary angiography

Is pulmonary angiography always necessary before treating a patient with a suspected PE?

No. If the clinical picture suggests PE, the chest x-ray is normal, and one or more mismatched segmental or subsegmental defects are present on a V/Q scan (i.e., a high probability scan), this is sufficient to continue treatment for a presumptive diagnosis of PE. However, pulmonary angiography is safe and allows easy consideration of some therapeutic options (filter, thrombolytic therapy).

When should a pulmonary angiogram be obtained?

To make a definitive diagnosis when the patient is at risk for complications from anticoagulation, or if the clinical picture is uncertain

What less invasive tests might be helpful in making the diagnosis?

In patients with low or intermediate probability scans, duplex scanning may demonstrate deep venous thrombosis (DVT) of the legs.

How high are the risks of major complications and death from pulmonary angiography?

Exceedingly low in the modern era

What are the initial supportive measures?

1. Supplemental oxygen
2. Mechanical ventilation (if required)
3. Intravenous access and fluid administration
4. Possibly vasopressors if the patient remains hypotensive

How is PE initially treated?

A 10,000–20,000 U bolus injection of IV heparin should be administered, followed by a continuous infusion of 1000–1500 U/hr. Minimal delay should occur in giving heparin after PE is suspected.

What laboratory tests should be obtained in monitoring heparin therapy?

A baseline partial thromboplastin time (PTT) should be obtained before initiation of heparin therapy, followed by additional measurements regularly to follow adequacy of anticoagulation. The heparin should be maintained at a rate that achieves a PTT of 1.5 to 2.0 times that of control values.

What is the major acute complication of heparin therapy?

Hemorrhage, but this is very rare with continuously infused heparin

Is the cancer patient at special risk for such complications?

The cancer patient may be at increased risk of bleeding due to thrombocytopenia from chemotherapy or antibiotics, or from known or unknown vascular invasion by neoplasm, from brain or epidural metastases, or gastrointestinal ulcerations.

Are there any absolute contraindications to anticoagulation?

Patients with known bleeding diatheses as well as patients with known neoplastic disease of the central nervous system should not be anticoagulated.

What can be done for such patients in the event of a PE?

In the case of massive or life-threatening PE, a sternotomy and pulmonary embolectomy may be required. Such patients require a vena caval filter or umbrella to prevent subsequent emboli.

What can be done for the patient who has failed anticoagulation therapy or who is at high risk from anticoagulant therapy?

Such patients are candidates for caval interruption procedures or vena caval filters.

Is surgical ligation of the inferior vena cava a common option?

No. Due to the morbidity and mortality rates of the procedure, especially in adults, it is very rarely, if ever, done.

Is pulmonary thromboembolectomy commonly performed?

No. Such patients with emboli massive enough to require this procedure often do not survive to reach the operating room.

What is the operative mortality rate of pulmonary thromboembolectomy?

About 50%

Is bowel obstruction a risk in the cancer patient?

Yes. Intestinal tumors are the third most common cause of intestinal obstruction.

What is the most common type of obstructing tumor?	Adenocarcinoma of the colon or rectum
How is bowel obstruction typically treated?	Initially, resuscitation involving making the patient NPO, administration of IV fluids, and insertion of a nasogastric tube. In the case of an obstructing tumor, this may be followed by resection of the tumor.
What is the most common cause of death in patients with metastatic cancer?	Organ failure from tumor invasion
Is bleeding a common cause of death in patients with cancer?	Yes. Bleeding is the third most common cause of cancer death in patients with metastatic cancer, following organ failure from tumor invasion and infection. It is the second most common cause of death in patients with hematologic neoplasms.
What are the most common causes of bleeding in the cancer patient?	Acute hemorrhagic gastritis, followed by peptic ulcer disease
What are some other causes of bleeding in the cancer patient?	Thrombocytopenia, abnormalities in plasma levels of coagulation factors, circulating inhibitory factors, and drugs
What types of drugs may cause bleeding and how?	Aspirin, other nonsteroidal analgesics, corticosteroids, chemotherapy, and antimicrobials can cause GI mucosal ulceration or may have direct effects on the level of platelets, their function, or on the circulating coagulation factors.
What is the most common cause of thrombocytopenia in the cancer patient?	Chemotherapy
Is acute life-threatening GI hemorrhage common in the cancer patient?	No. Most episodes of bleeding are minor and not of hemodynamic significance.

Acute life-threatening GI hemorrhage in the cancer patient results from what?

Hemorrhage can occur as a result of hemostatic abnormalities or structural pathology such as mucosal chemotoxicity, radiation enteritis, or erosions and ulcerations due to neoplasm or infection.

Which types of neoplasms are most commonly associated with upper GI bleeding when bleeding is due directly to the neoplasm?

Gastric lymphoma, gastric leiomyosarcoma, and gastric carcinoma

Is gastric carcinoma a common cause of upper GI bleeding?

No. It accounts for only about 5% of all upper GI bleeding.

What are some other, less common, causes of acute upper GI bleeding in the cancer patient?

Mallory-Weiss syndrome, esophageal varices secondary to cirrhosis and portal hypertension or to massive hepatic replacement by tumor or acute portal vein thrombosis, acute erosive fungal or viral esophagitis, and biliary tract hemorrhage

How is the Mallory-Weiss syndrome related to the cancer patient?

Several authors have reported Mallory-Weiss syndrome in cancer patients with chemotherapy-induced vomiting.

In patients presenting with massive lower GI bleeding, what percentage are due to a cancer or polyp?

About 10%

Define massive hemoptysis.

Expectoration of at least 600 ml of blood in a 24-hour period, or intrabronchial bleeding at such a rate as to present a threat to life

Do patients with massive hemoptysis usually die of exsanguination?

No. The actual cause of death is usually flooding of the bronchial tree with blood causing asphyxiation by interference with gas exchange.

What is the most common cause of massive hemoptysis in patients over the age of 40?

Bronchogenic carcinoma

Patients with which histologic type of bronchogenic carcinoma are most likely to present with massive hemoptysis?

Squamous cell (epidermoid) carcinoma

What procedure should all patients with massive hemoptysis undergo to determine the site and cause of bleeding?

Bronchoscopy

Which type of bronchoscopy is considered the technique of choice?

Traditionally, rigid bronchoscopy has been the technique of choice for evaluation of massive hemoptysis because of its larger diameter and its better ability to suction, administer oxygen, and control the airway. Rigid bronchoscopy requires general anesthesia and does not allow visualization of the upper lobe bronchi. Flexible bronchoscopy has become more popular recently because of its lack of requirement for general anesthesia and its ability to inspect a much larger area of the bronchial tree. Difficulty in suctioning large amounts of blood and maintaining oxygenation are its drawbacks.

What is the initial treatment for massive hemoptysis?

Once the bleeding site is identified, the patient is placed bleeding side down to avoid aspiration into the nonbleeding lung. Oxygen, intravenous fluids, and blood products are given as appropriate. Selective bronchial intubation may be performed to protect the patient's airway, and a balloon catheter (Fogarty) may be passed through the rigid bronchoscope to tamponade the bleeding site.

What is the definitive treatment of massive hemoptysis?

Surgical resection of the bleeding pulmonary segment

What is the mortality rate of conservative, nonsurgical management?

50%–100%. Therefore, a thoracic surgical consult should be obtained in all cases of massive hemoptysis.

What options exist for patients who are not surgical candidates?

Prolonged balloon tamponade with a Fogarty catheter and arteriography with therapeutic embolization of bronchial (not pulmonary) arteries. Radiation therapy may be helpful in controlling bleeding tumors, but an effect may be delayed by several days.

Which malignancies commonly produce malignant pleural effusions?

Carcinomas of the lung and breast as well as lymphomas

What is the pathophysiology of a malignant pleural effusion?

Decreased lymphatic outflow secondary to malignant obstruction and increased capillary permeability resulting in an exudative effusion

What are the treatment options for patients with malignant pleural effusions?

Tube thoracostomy with chemical pleurodesis, thoracoscopy with talc pleurodesis, and rarely pleurectomy or pleuroperitoneal shunt

Does the development of a pleural effusion necessarily signify incurable disease?

In most circumstances, the development of an effusion signifies advanced, incurable disease. However, with certain malignancies such as lymphoma, the patient may still be effectively treated and even cured of disease even if a true malignant effusion is present.

What "remote" effects of a neoplasm may result in pleural effusion?

Hypoproteinemia, mediastinal lymphatic obstruction, superior vena caval obstruction, pericardial tamponade

What else should be considered in the differential diagnosis?

Congestive heart failure, fluid overload, pneumonitis, tuberculosis, PE, autoimmune disease, and drug toxicity

What chemotherapeutic agents have been implicated as causing pleural effusions?	Methotrexate, procarbazine, cyclophosphamide, mitomycin, and bleomycin
What are common symptoms of malignant pleural effusions?	Dyspnea, orthopnea, cough, and chest pain
To what aspect of the effusions are symptoms most closely related?	Symptoms appear to be more closely related to the rate of fluid accumulation than to the total volume.
How often are malignant pleural effusions bilateral?	About 1/3 of patients have bilateral effusions.
What is the most common cause of massive pleural effusion (> 2 L)?	Cancer
How is the diagnosis of pleural effusion made?	Initially by physical exam with decreased breath sounds and dullness to percussion over the affected area. The diagnosis is then confirmed by chest x-ray.
Blunting of the costophrenic angle represents how much pleural fluid?	300–500 ml of pleural fluid
What specific x-ray is useful in cases where the diagnosis is in question or in cases of subpulmonic effusion?	The lateral decubitus chest x-ray is useful here, detecting as little as 100 ml of pleural fluid.
How is the diagnosis of malignant pleural effusion typically made?	By thoracentesis and cytology
Which patients should undergo therapeutic thoracentesis?	Patients with significant dyspnea, hypoxemia, mediastinal shift, hemodynamic instability, or evidence of empyema should undergo thoracentesis promptly.

Total drainage during the first 12 hours should not exceed about 1500 ml. Why?

This is done to avoid the risk of unilateral expansion PE, due to rapid changes in pressure gradients.

What is the survival of patients with malignant pleural effusions at 6 months?

The overall prognosis is poor. The survival at 6 months is less than 25%. Survival is slightly better in patients with lymphoma and breast cancer.

What are the most common GI problems requiring operation in patients with cancer?

Obstruction, hemorrhage, and perforation

What is the most common cause of bowel obstruction in cancer patients?

Primary or metastatic malignancy, followed by benign causes such as adhesions and radiation enteritis (as opposed to the predominantly benign causes of obstruction seen in the overall population with bowel obstruction)

What are the most common sources of GI bleeding in patients with cancer?

Peptic ulcer disease and gastritis, often exacerbated by thrombocytopenia, coagulopathy, and corticosteroid use. Hemorrhage from tumors is less common.

What are some factors resulting in the syndromes of ileus and pseudo-obstruction in oncology patients?

Narcotics, anticholinergic medications (e.g., many antiemetics), chemotherapeutic agents (particularly vincristine), electrolyte imbalance, and tumor-related disruption of autonomic supply

Describe the clinical syndrome of neutropenic enterocolitis.

Neutropenic enterocolitis, also known as typhlitis, affects patients who are neutropenic from chemotherapy, generally in the setting of hematologic malignancy. It consists of febrile neutropenia, abdominal pain (principally right lower quadrant), distention, and diarrhea. The diagnosis is one of exclusion, and CT findings of bowel wall thickening affecting the ileum and right colon often with pneumatosis are helpful but are inconstant and nonspecific.

What is the treatment of neutropenic enterocolitis?

Complete bowel rest with total parenteral nutrition and broad spectrum antibiotics. Indications for surgery include progressive symptoms, sepsis, hemorrhage, or perforation. Surgery generally requires right hemicolectomy and ileostomy.

Describe the types of "permanent" central venous catheters commonly used in cancer patients.

1. Tunneled, external, cuffed, dual, or single lumen catheters such as the Hickman, Broviac, Leonard, or Groshong catheters
2. Implantable ports, dual or single lumen, such as the port-a-cath

What is the difference between Hickman-type (Hickman, Broviac, Leonard, etc.) and Groshong central venous catheters?

Hickman-type catheters have no valves, require a daily flush and heparin lock, and are excellent for repeated infusions of blood products. Groshong catheters have a slit-valve end, allowing less frequent flushing and elimination of the heparin lock, and are less suitable for frequent blood product infusions. There is no significant difference in patency or infection rates between the two types.

What is the syndrome of cancer cachexia?

Cancer cachexia is the catabolic state present in many cancer patients that is believed to be secondary to tumor-host interactions resulting in the release of cytokines, particularly TNF and interleukin-6. It consists of weight loss, anorexia, muscle wasting, weakness, hyperlipidemia, glucose intolerance, and hepatic gluconeogenesis despite adequate intake of protein and calories.

What is SIADH?

The syndrome of inappropriate ADH secretion, resulting in hypervolemic hyponatremia. Findings include hyponatremia with an inappropriately high urine sodium, and a urine osmolality greater than that of the plasma.

What is the most common malignancy associated with SIADH?

Small-cell lung cancer

What is the treatment of SIADH?

Severe hyponatremia should be treated with normal saline and furosemide with a slow (< 1 mEq/l/hr) correction in sodium. The overall treatment is directed at the treatment of the primary cancer. Otherwise, the first line therapy is free water restriction. Demeclocycline, an ADH antagonist, can be used in resistant cases.

What are some mechanisms of tumor-related hypoglycemia?

1. Insulin production by insulinomas
2. Production of insulin-like peptides such as IGF-1, IGF-2, and somatomedins by tumors such as hepatocellular carcinomas, some sarcomas, and mesotheliomas

What is the most common complaint in patients with malignant spinal cord compression?

Pain, generally exacerbated by movement, coughing, or valsalva. The majority of patients also have weakness, sensory deficits, and autonomic dysfunction.

Section 4

Patient-Specific Considerations in the ICU

21

Pediatric Patients

AIRWAY

What are the signs of respiratory distress in infants and children?

Tachypnea, stridor, grunting, nasal flaring, retraction of the chest wall, and cyanosis. As in all age groups, much of what you will learn about a child's respiratory status can be observed by watching the movement of the chest wall.

What are appropriate-sized endotracheal tubes for infants and children?

1. Premature infant: 2.5–3.0 mm
2. Infant: 3.0–3.5 mm
3. Toddler: 4.0–4.5 mm
4. Young school-aged child: 5.0–5.5 mm
5. Older children: 6.0–7.0 mm

What are the two methods of estimating the appropriate-sized endotracheal tube for an infant or child?

1. Infant: tube diameter equals nostril or the smallest finger
2. Child: $\dfrac{(16 + \text{age in years})}{4}$

When are cuffed endotracheal tubes used?

Usually only in children beyond the toddler and preschool years

Why are cuffs avoided in infants and toddlers?

To avoid trauma to the airway and subsequent subglottic stenosis. This is especially true in premature and term infants.

How long may premature and term infants be intubated with an endotracheal tube?

Almost indefinitely with adherence to these principles:
1. Appropriate-sized uncuffed tube
2. Tube should allow leak around it at 20 cm H_2O positive pressure.
3. Securing of endotracheal tube so it does not move, to avoid airway traumas

When are tracheostomies used?

Essentially never in premature infants. Infants may require a tracheostomy in cases of long-term airway access needed secondary to neurologic damage or congenital defects (e.g., severe micrognathia or cleft palate). Older children usually will need tracheostomies for long-term care in cases of severe neurologic damage from primary disease or trauma.

What is the first step in resuscitation of a child with a tracheostomy who has respiratory distress?

The tracheostomy should be examined for patency and appropriate position. Because of the small size of a child's airway, children are especially vulnerable to mucous plugging and malposition of tracheostomies.

What are important anatomic considerations in maintaining an airway in infants?

1. An infant has a large head predisposing to neck flexion. Keep extension maintained until the endotracheal tube is placed.
2. Larynx is more caudad than in older children.
3. Mask ventilation.

What procedure do you perform to provide an airway for a child who has significant facial trauma?

A needle cricothyroidotomy. A 14-gauge or 16-gauge needle may be used and connected to a jet ventilator.

What is the most likely cause of right upper lobe lung collapse in a child maintained on mechanical ventilation?

Right mainstem bronchus intubation or edema at the right upper lobe (RUL) branch secondary to an endotracheal tube being too low in the trachea. The trachea in children is very short and the appropriate placement of the tip of the endotracheal tube has a range of about 1 cm in children younger than age 4.

What side effects does prolonged high oxygen content administered during mechanical ventilation have on infants (especially premature infants)?

1. Bronchopulmonary dysplasia (a type of fibrosis)
2. Retrolental fibroplasia (retinal damage)

Is it appropriate to wait to perform cardiac countershock in a child who has arrested?	Yes. Unlike advanced life support in adults, resuscitation of an asystolic child involves a trial of ventilation with 100% oxygen before cardiac countershock is performed.
What complication following general anesthesia is especially worrisome in babies younger than 50 weeks' gestational age?	Apneic episodes. For this reason, elective surgeries are postponed until the age of 50 weeks, or the child is admitted to the hospital for ECG and pulse oximetry monitoring postoperatively.

STRIDOR

What is stridor?	Harsh noise heard on breathing caused by obstruction of the trachea or larynx; often accounted for in the newborn by congenital malformations causing airway obstruction.
Symptoms and signs?	1. Dyspnea 2. Cyanosis 3. Difficulty with feedings
Differential diagnosis?	1. Laryngomalacia—#1 cause of stridor in the infant. Results from inadequate development of supporting structures of the larynx. Usually self-limited and treatment is expectant unless respiratory compromise is present. 2. Tracheobronchomalacia—similar to laryngomalacia, but involves entire trachea 3. Vascular rings and slings—abnormal development or position of thoracic large vessels resulting in obstruction of trachea/bronchus
Symptoms of vascular rings?	1. Stridor 2. Dyspnea on exertion 3. Dysphagia
How are vascular rings diagnosed?	1. Barium swallow revealing typical configuration of esophageal compression 2. Echo/arteriogram

How are vascular rings treated?	Surgical division of ring if the patient is symptomatic

ECMO

What does ECMO stand for?	Extracorporeal membrane oxygenation
What is it and what does it do?	It is a form of cardiopulmonary bypass. It provides an external membrane for oxygenating blood independent of native lung function.
What are indications for ECMO therapy?	The most frequent use of ECMO is in the neonatal population. Indications have included meconium aspiration, sepsis, diaphragmatic hernias, pneumonia, and cardiac failure. A heterogeneous group of diseases are treated with ECMO. The criteria used to determine the need for ECMO vary from hospital to hospital, but such criteria should predict an 80%–90% mortality rate if ECMO were not used.
How does ECMO work?	A central artery and vein are cannulated. The right common carotid artery and the right internal jugular vein are the vessels most commonly used in children. The baby's blood volume is then pumped past an oxygenating membrane and warmer. Systemic heparinization must be maintained to prevent clotting. This provides respiratory support for days to 2–4 weeks, allowing the original problem to resolve.

SHOCK

What is the definition of shock?	Inadequate end-organ perfusion
What is appropriate urine output for infants and children?	1. Infant: 2 ml/kg/hr 2. Toddler: 1–2 ml/kg/hr 3. School-aged child: 1 ml/kg/hr 4. Adolescent: 1/2 ml/kg/hr

What are maintenance fluid requirements for infants and small children?

1. 100 ml/kg/day for the first 10 kg; 50 ml/kg/day for the next 10 kg; 25 ml/kg/day for each 10 kg after
2. This may be calculated by the "4,2,1" rule: 4 ml/kg/hr for the first 10 kg; 2 ml/kg/hr for the next 10 kg; 1 ml/kg/hr for each 10 kg after.

What is important to remember about the infant's and child's cardiovascular response to hypovolemia?

Adequate blood pressure will be maintained until about 25% of volume is lost! Tachycardia and decreased urine output are earlier signs of hypovolemia.

What causes shock?

Hypovolemia (especially trauma, severe enteritis), spinal cord injury, cardiac failure, sepsis, and anaphylaxis

How does a child's fluid resuscitation needs differ from an adult's and why?

Children have a relatively greater total body water content than adults. Most of this is contained in extracellular fluid. Renal function in childhood is also less efficient, and children are less able to concentrate their urine, thus wasting electrolytes and water during periods of dehydration. These factors make children less able to tolerate fluid and electrolyte losses.

At what rate should fluids be replaced?

In 20 ml/kg boluses until adequate urine output is obtained.

What types of intravenous fluids are recommended for repletion and maintenance of intravascular volume in children?

Lactated Ringer's is the closest crystalloid solution to the composition of blood and is used for fluid boluses. Because renal function is less mature in infants, 50% normal saline (NS) is sometimes used in smaller quantities for resuscitation to avoid acute sodium and fluid overload. D5 0.25% NS with 20 mEq KCl is recommended for maintenance fluids.

What routes of vascular access are available in pediatric patients that are not available in adult patients?

Intraosseous venous access and access to umbilical vessels

How and when is an intraosseous line placed?	Intraosseous lines are most frequently placed in the proximal, medial tibia. A sturdy 16-gauge or 18-gauge needle is most often used. This allows access to the bone marrow that drains into the venous system. This type of access is useful in patients younger than the age of 8 years who are severely volume depleted and in whom placement of any other peripheral intravenous line is not possible.
How long may an intraosseous line stay in place?	No longer than 6 hours
Central lines are placed using what type of technique in premature or small-for-gestational-age infants?	Venous cutdown techniques are used to place central access in small babies.
Why do premature infants have even greater water requirements than term infants?	Their skin is extremely thin, which allows potentially twice the insensible loss of water that would normally be expected for their surface area.
What amount of blood is normally given to pediatric patients when they need a transfusion?	10 ml/kg

NECROTIZING ENTEROCOLITIS (NEC)

What is NEC?	Necrosis of intestinal mucosa, often with bleeding; may progress to transmural intestinal necrosis, shock/sepsis, and death
Predisposing conditions?	Stress: shock, hypoxia, respiratory distress syndrome, apneic episodes, sepsis, exchange transfusions, patent ductus arteriosus and cyanotic heart disease, hyperosmolar feedings, polycythemia, indomethacin treatment

Pathophysiologic mechanism?	Probable splanchnic vasoconstriction with decreased perfusion, mucosal injury, and probably bacterial invasion
What is NEC's claim to infamy?	Most common cause of emergent laparotomy in the neonate
Signs and symptoms?	Abdominal distention, vomiting, heme + or gross rectal bleeding, fever or hypothermia, jaundice, abdominal wall erythema (consistent with perforation and abscess formation)
Radiographic findings?	Fixed, dilated intestinal loops, pneumatosis intestinalis (air in the bowel wall), free air, and portal vein air (sign of advanced disease)
Laboratory findings?	Low hematocrit, low glucose, low platelets
Treatment?	3/4 managed medically: 1. Cessation of enteral feedings 2. Orogastric tube 3. IV fluids/total parenteral nutrition (TPN) 4. IV antibiotics 5. Ventilator support as needed
Surgical indications?	Free air in abdomen revealing perforation and positive peritoneal tap revealing transmural bowel necrosis.
Indications for peritoneal tap?	Severe thrombocytopenia, distended abdomen, abdominal wall erythema, unexplained clinical downturn in the face of maximal medical therapy
Complications?	Occur commonly and include further bowel necrosis, gram-negative sepsis, disseminated intravascular coagulopathy, wound infection, cholestasis, short bowel syndrome, strictures, and late small bowel obstruction
Prognosis?	Greater than 80% overall survival

MISCELLANEOUS

What does bilious vomiting in an infant signify?	Malrotation with volvulus until proven otherwise! About 90% of patients with malrotation present with bilious vomiting before their first year of life. Immediate diagnostic study should be done.
How is malrotation diagnosed?	Abnormally placed ligament of Treitz on upper GI
What does TORCHES stand for?	Nonbacterial fetal and neonatal infection: **TO**xoplasmosis, **R**ubella, **C**ytomegalovirus (CMV), **HE**rpes, **S**yphilis
Signs of child abuse?	Cigarette burns, rope burns, scald to posterior thighs and buttocks, multiple fractures/old fractures, genital trauma, delay in accessing health care system
How are chest compressions performed in children?	For infants and toddlers younger than age 1, one to two fingers are used to compress the sternum. The rate of compressions is from 100–120 per minute. The depth of compressions is adequate when a palpable pulse over the brachial artery is obtained. Five compressions are done for each breath administered. For children younger than age 10, one hand is used for compressions, and a rate of 100 compressions per minute is the goal.
Why are infants and children so prone to becoming hypothermic?	They have a greater body surface area-to-volume ratio so that more heat escapes through their skin. They also have a lower percentage of body fat to help insulate against heat loss.
What measures are taken to prevent this loss of heat?	The infant's or child's ambient temperature is kept appropriate with incubators, warming lights, operating room temperature, and blankets. Care is taken to reduce exposure of abdominal or thoracic cavity contents for protracted periods, and IV fluids and ventilator gases are warmed before administration.

At what weight can an infant begin to self-regulate its body temperature?

About 1800–2000 g

Do healthy children have different nutritional needs than adults, and if so, why?

Yes, children have tremendous metabolic needs. This is caused by rapid cell division and growth. They also have fewer nutritional reserves in the form of fat.

What are the baseline nutritional requirements of children?

Infants need 110 kcal/kg/day, and this need gradually decreases to 40 kcal/kg/day in adulthood.

What routes are available to feed children who cannot eat?

Peripheral parenteral nutrition (PPN), TPN, and enteral tube feedings. These routes are very similar to those available for adults, including modes of access and types of complications that may result.

22

Trauma Patients

Trauma care in the United States follows what widely accepted protocol?

The Advanced Trauma Life Support (ATLS) precepts of the American College of Surgeons.

What is the brief ATLS history?

An **"AMPLE"** history:
Allergies
Medications
PMH
Last meal (when)
Events (of injury, etc.)

What are the three main elements of the ATLS protocol?

1. Primary survey/resuscitation
2. Secondary survey
3. Definitive care

What about the patient history?

This should be obtained while completing the primary survey. Often, the rescue squad, witnesses, and family members must be relied upon.

PRIMARY SURVEY

What are the five steps of the primary survey? (You *must* know these!)
A?

Airway

B?

Breathing

C?

Circulation

D?

Disability

E?

Exposure

What principles are followed in completing the primary survey?

Life-threatening problems discovered during the primary survey are always addressed before proceeding to the next step.

AIRWAY

What are the goals during assessment of the airway?	Securing the airway and protecting the spinal cord.
In addition to the airway, what must be considered during the airway step?	Spinal immobilization if there is any question of spinal injury.
What constitutes adequate spinal immobilization?	Use of a full backboard and rigid cervical collar.
In an alert patient, what is the quickest test for an adequate airway?	Ask a question. If the patient can speak, the airway is intact.
What is the first maneuver used to establish an airway?	Chin lift and/or jaw thrust. If successful, often an oral or nasal airway can be used to temporarily maintain the airway.
If these methods are unsuccessful, what is the next maneuver used to establish an airway?	Endotracheal intubation via either the nasal or oral route.
Contraindication to nasotracheal intubation?	Maxillofacial fracture!
If all other methods are unsuccessful, how should an emergent airway be established?	Cricothyroidotomy, either by percutaneous placement of a needle through the cricothyroid membrane or by surgical placement of a tube through the cricothyroid membrane ("surgical airway").
What must always be kept in mind during difficult attempts at establishing an airway?	Spinal immobilization and adequate oxygenation. If at all possible, patients must be adequately ventilated with 100% oxygen using a bag and mask before any attempt at establishing an airway.

BREATHING

What are the goals in assessing breathing?	Securing oxygenation and ventilation and treatment of life-threatening thoracic injuries.

What comprises adequate assessment of breathing?

1. Inspection: for air movement, respiratory rate, cyanosis, tracheal shift, jugular venous distention, asymmetric chest expansion, use of accessory muscles of respiration, open chest wounds
2. Auscultation: for upper airway sounds (stridor, wheezing, or gurgling), and for lower airway sounds present over both lung fields
3. Percussion: hyperresonance or dullness over either lung field
4. Palpation: presence of subcutaneous emphysema, flail segments

What are six life-threatening conditions that must be diagnosed and treated during the breathing step?

1. Airway obstruction
2. Tension pneumothorax
3. Open pneumothorax
4. Flail chest
5. Cardiac tamponade
6. Massive hemothorax

How is a pneumothorax diagnosed?

Dyspnea, tachypnea, anxiety, pleuritic chest pain, unilateral decreased or absent breath sounds, tracheal shift away from the affected side, hyperresonance on the affected side. Remember, tension pneumothorax is a clinical diagnosis not a radiologic diagnosis!

What is the treatment for a pneumothorax?

Immediate decompression by needle thoracostomy in the second intercostal space, midclavicular line, followed by tube thoracostomy placed in the anterior/midaxillary line in the fourth intercostal space (level of the nipple in males).

How is an open pneumothorax, also known as sucking chest wound, diagnosed?

Usually obvious, with air movement through a chest wall defect.

How is this open wound treated?

In the ER: intubation with positive-pressure ventilation, tube thoracostomy (chest tube), occlusive dressing.

Why is an open pneumothorax a potentially lethal injury?

If the chest wall defect is greater than two thirds of the diameter of the trachea, air will preferentially enter the chest through the defect rather than the airway during inspiration and the patient will be unable to breathe.

How is flail chest diagnosed?

The "classic" picture is that of four or more multiply fractured ribs resulting in a segment of chest wall that moves paradoxically and results in immediate hypoventilation. (The real culprit in this scenario is the almost inevitable underlying pulmonary contusion that results in progressive respiratory failure.)

How is flail chest treated?

Intubation with positive pressure ventilation and positive end-expiratory pressure (PEEP).

How is pulmonary contusion treated?

Restrict intravenous fluids. Avoid colloid. Positive pressure ventilation is often needed.

How is cardiac tamponade diagnosed?

Beck's triad of decreased heart sounds, jugular venous distention, and decreased blood pressure. (Full triad is present in only one third of patients with this diagnosis.) Also, tachycardia, pulsus paradoxus, Kussmaul's signs. Hypotension due to tamponade implies imminent cardiac collapse. Note: this entity is very rare with blunt trauma but common with penetrating trauma.

How is cardiac tamponade treated?

Immediate IV fluid bolus and pericardiocentesis. Subsequent surgical exploration is mandatory. If patient's stability will allow it, a subxiphoid pericardial window is the preferred diagnostic test.

How is massive hemothorax diagnosed?

Hypotension, unilaterally decreased or absent breath sounds, dullness to percussion; obvious on chest x-ray if massive (but remember up to 500 ml of blood can be hidden by the diaphragm on upright chest x-ray).

How is massive hemothorax treated?	Volume replacement, tube thoracostomy (large chest tube); use a cell saver if available; removal of the blood will allow apposition of the parietal and visceral pleura, which will often seal the defect and slow the bleeding.

CIRCULATION

What are the goals in assessing circulation?	1. Securing adequate tissue perfusion 2. Treating external bleeding
What is the initial test for adequate circulation?	Palpation of pulses; as a rough guide, if a femoral or carotid pulse is palpable, then systolic pressure is at least 60 mm Hg; if a radial pulse is palpable, then systolic pressure is at least 80 mm Hg.
What comprises adequate assessment of circulation?	Heart rate, blood pressure, peripheral perfusion (e.g., capillary refill, skin temperature), urinary output, mental status. (Beware of relying only on the blood pressure, especially in the young patient in whom autonomic tone can maintain blood pressure until cardiovascular collapse is imminent.)
What signs are suggestive of poor tissue perfusion upon examination of the skin?	Capillary refill more than 2 seconds. Cold, clammy skin.
How are sites of external bleeding treated?	By direct pressure. Avoid tourniquets and blind clamping of bleeding sites, as both lead to increased limb loss.
What is the preferred intravenous access in the trauma patient?	Two large-bore (14–16 gauge) IV catheters in the upper extremities.
What are the alternate sites of IV access?	Percutaneous and cutdown catheters in the lower leg saphenous (cutdown) and femoral veins (percutaneous); avoid subclavian and jugular lines if possible because of the increased morbidity of placement and the smaller diameter of the catheters.

How does one remember the anatomy of the groin for insertion of a femoral vein catheter?	**NAVEL** (from lateral to medial): **N**erve; **A**rtery; **V**ein; **E**mpty space; **L**igaments. Thus, the vein is medial to the femoral artery pulse.
What is the resuscitation fluid of choice in trauma patients?	Lactated Ringer's solution, which is isotonic; the lactate helps buffer the hypovolemia-induced metabolic acidosis.
Why is normal saline not as appealing?	The high chloride content causes a dilutional acidosis by diluting out the serum bicarbonate.
What types of hollow organ decompression must the trauma patient receive?	Gastric decompression with a nasogastric (NG) tube and Foley catheter bladder decompression after a normal rectal exam.
In the presence of a maxillofacial fracture, how should gastric decompression be accomplished?	NOT with an NG tube, as the tube may perforate the cribriform plate and move into the brain if maxillofacial fracture/skull fracture is present. Place an orogastric tube (OGT), not an NG tube.

DISABILITY

What are the goals in assessing disability?	Determination of neurologic injury. (Think neurologic disability.)
What comprises adequate assessment of disability?	1. Mental status: Glasgow Coma Scale (GCS) 2. Pupils: a blown pupil reflects an intracranial mass lesion (blood) as CN III is compressed (mass lesion is on the same side as blown pupil 90% of the time) 3. Motor/sensory: screening exam for extremity movement, sensation

EXPOSURE

What are the goals in obtaining adequate exposure?	Complete disrobing to allow a thorough visual inspection and digital palpation of the patient during the secondary survey.

SECONDARY SURVEY

What principle is followed in completing the secondary survey?	Complete physical examination including all orifices: ears, nose, mouth, vagina, rectum.

Why look in the ears?

Hemotympanum and otorrhea are signs of a basilar skull fracture.

Examination of what part of the trauma patient's body is often forgotten?

The patient's back—logroll the patient and examine! (Especially pertinent in penetrating trauma.)

What are the typical signs of a basilar skull fracture?

Raccoon eyes, Battle's sign (mastoid hematoma), clear otorrhea or rhinorrhea, hemotympanum

What sign of an anterior chamber bleeding must not be missed on the eye exam?

Traumatic hyphema

What potentially destructive lesion must not be missed on the nasal exam?

Nasal septal hematoma; if left unevacuated, the hematoma will result in pressure necrosis of the septum.

What is the best indication of a mandibular fracture?

Dental malocclusion. As the patient bites down, ask, "Does that feel normal to you?"

What signs of thoracic trauma are often found on the neck exam?

Crepitus or subcutaneous emphysema from tracheobronchial disruption, tracheal deviation from tension pneumothorax, jugular venous distention from cardiac tamponade, carotid bruit heard with carotid artery injury from seatbelt trauma

What is the best exam for broken ribs or sternum?

Lateral and anterior-posterior compression of the thorax to elicit pain

What physical signs are diagnostic for thoracic great vessel injury?

None: diagnosis of great vessel injury requires a high index of suspicion based on mechanism of injury, associated injuries, and chest x-ray/radiographic findings.

What must be considered in every penetrating injury of the thorax at or below the level of the nipple?

Concomitant injury to the abdomen. Remember, the diaphragm rises to the level of the nipples in males on full expiration.

What is the proper technique for examining the thoracic and lumbar spine?

Logrolling the patient to allow complete visualization of the back and palpation of the spine to elicit pain or detect a deformity over a fracture.

What conditions must exist to pronounce an abdominal physical exam normal?

An alert patient without any evidence of head/spinal cord injury, drug/ethyl alcohol intoxication, or distracting injuries elsewhere in the body.

What physical signs may indicate intra-abdominal injury?

Guarding, tenderness, rebound tenderness, and other signs of peritoneal irritation, progressive distension, absent bowel sounds

What must be documented from the rectal exam?

1. Sphincter tone as an indication of spinal cord injury
2. Presence of blood as an indication of colon or rectal injury
3. Prostate position as an indication of urethral injury

What is the best technique to use for detection of pelvic and hip fractures?

Lateral compression of the iliac crests and greater trochanters and anterior-posterior compression of the symphysis pubis to elicit pain

What four physical signs indicate possible urethral injury, thus contraindicating placement of a Foley catheter?

1. High-riding, ballottable prostate on rectal exam
2. Presence of blood at the penile meatus
3. Scrotal or perineal ecchymosis
4. Inability of the patient to spontaneously void

What must be documented from the extremity exam?

Any fractures or joint injuries, any open wounds, motor and sensory exam particularly distal to any fractures, distal pulses, and peripheral perfusion

What complication is often seen after prolonged ischemia to an extremity that must be treated immediately to save the extremity, and what is that treatment?

Compartment syndrome, treated by fasciotomies

What injuries must be suspected in a trauma patient with a progressive decline in mental status?	Epidural hematoma, subdural hematoma, cerebral edema with rising intracranial pressure. One must also rule out hypoxia/hypotension.

MISCELLANEOUS TRAUMA FACTS

What is the lowest acceptable urine output for an adult trauma patient?	50 ml/hr
What findings would require a celiotomy in a blunt trauma victim?	Peritoneal signs, free air on abdominal x-ray, positive diagnostic peritoneal lavage, evidence of certain injuries on CT scan.
How much blood can be lost into the thigh with a closed femur fracture?	Up to 3 L of blood, or more than half the patient's blood volume!
Can an adult lose enough blood in the skull from a brain injury to cause hypovolemic shock?	Absolutely NOT! However, infants can lose enough blood from a brain injury to cause shock, as their fontanelles have not yet closed and the skull can expand.
What are some signs of adequate fluid resuscitation in the trauma patient?	Resolving tachycardia, adequate urine output, resolving acidosis, warm and pink extremities (adequate peripheral perfusion)
What is oxygen delivery (DO_2) and how is it measured?	Oxygen delivery is the amount of oxygen delivered to peripheral tissues. It is measured in ml/min and is determined from the following formula: DO_2 = cardiac output × hemoglobin × 1.34 (conversion factor for oxygen carrying capacity of hemoglobin) × oxygen saturation (0.0–1.0). Optimal value is controversial but should be greater than 500 ml/min. Normal = 1000.
Coagulopathy and low filling pressures after laparotomy for trauma indicate what process?	Continued bleeding. It is often impossible to correct coagulopathy in the face of continued traumatic hemorrhage. Reexploration is often necessary.

What is the work-up for fever in the ICU patient after trauma?

Chest x-ray, CBC with differential, urine analysis and culture, appropriate tests including thorough physical exam and the review of pertinent history. Always change or remove indwelling lines, especially those with sugar in them. (Arterial lines almost never cause infection.)

Should endotracheal tubes be removed from the nasal passages of chronic ICU patients?

Yes. These tubes often impede drainage from the sinuses leading to stasis and bacterial infection. This is a source of infection that must be investigated in the trauma victim. Large NG tubes should also be replaced as early as possible with feeding tubes.

Which type of feeding decreases infectious complication in ICU trauma patients?

Enteral feeding has been shown to decrease nosocomial pneumonia, ICU days, and ventilator days after trauma. Total parenteral nutrition (TPN) has an increased rate of sepsis compared to enteral feeding. (Remember: start slowly. The lungs are a very poor place for food to be absorbed.)

What is abdominal compartment syndrome?

This can occur after major trauma. It is characterized by increased intra-abdominal pressure due to blood in the abdomen, gas in the bowel, bowel wall edema, or edema or blood in the retroperitoneum. This increased pressure decreases renal and intestinal blood flow as well as decreases pulmonary compliance and worsens respiratory status.

How is abdominal compartment pressure measured?

With a Foley catheter. 100 ml of fluid is instilled in the bladder through the sampling port, and the catheter tubing is filled with fluid. The tubing is then clamped distal to the port, and the port is entered with a needle connected to a calibrated pressure transducer and the intra-abdominal pressure is measured. A value greater than 25 mm Hg requires decompression of the abdomen.

What is the treatment for abdominal compartment syndrome?

Open the abdomen. There are many techniques described to deal with the abdominal cavity. One is the "vac pac" technique. The bowel is placed in a bowel bag and covered with moist towels. Two Jackson-Pratt drains are placed over the towels and then a large Ioban drape is placed over the entire abdomen after prepping the skin with Benzoin. The drains are then connected to high wall suction.

At what point should tracheostomy be performed in the trauma ICU patient?

This is controversial. However, there is general consensus that early tracheostomy decreases ventilator days, mortality, and allows for easier ventilator weaning. Tracheostomy is probably indicated if the patient is ventilated for at least 10 days or has failed extubation twice. Some say that a tracheostomy is almost always overdue by the time the clinician has thought of it.

Is it important to complete all diagnostic studies before admitting a trauma patient to the ICU?

No. Patients can be better warmed and more closely monitored in the ICU setting. It is usually in the patient's best interest to be moved to the ICU as soon as the need for surgery has been excluded.

Ten days after a splenectomy, a trauma patient develops fever, leukocytosis, and left upper quadrant pain. What is the likely diagnosis?

Subphrenic abscess

What are some laboratory tests that indicate poor perfusion?

Elevated lactate. Lactate value trends are probably better indicators than examining single values. High mortality is reported for patients with lactate greater than 2 mg/dl, 24 hours after admission.

What are more invasive methods used to determine adequate resuscitation from trauma?

The Swan-Ganz catheter is used to measure cardiac output and mixed venous oxygen saturation.

In what population is a surgical cricothyroidotomy NOT recommended?	Any patient younger than 12 years old. (Instead perform needle cricothyroidotomy.)
What are common intra-abdominal injuries associated with seatbelt use?	Intestinal injuries, fracture of second lumbar vertebra, and pancreatic injury

ORTHOPEDIC TRAUMA

COMPARTMENT SYNDROME

What is a compartment syndrome?	Increase in intracompartmental pressure of an extremity with associated neurovascular compromise
Etiology?	1. Fractures 2. Tight fascial surgical closure 3. Tight cast/bandage application 4. Increased third-space fluid secondary to ischemic/reperfusion injury or burns 5. Crush injury 6. Electrical injury
Injuries with high incidence of extremity compartment syndrome?	1. Burns and electrical injuries 2. Supracondylar elbow fractures (especially in children) 3. Proximal tibial fractures
Compartments in the lower leg?	1. Lateral 2. Anterior 3. Posterior-superficial 4. Posterior-deep
Compartments in the forearm?	1. Extensor 2. Flexor-superficial 3. Flexor-deep
Other compartments in the body?	1. Skull 2. Pericardium 3. Chest 4. Abdomen

What tissues cause the compression phenomenon of compartment syndromes?	1. Fascia 2. Skin 3. Bone
Signs/symptoms of extremity compartment syndrome?	The six **P**s: 1. **P**ain out of proportion to injury, especially with passive flexion/extension; usually earliest indicator 2. **P**ulselessness; inconsistent. May have a pulse with a compartment syndrome. Loss of pulses is last effect of increasing compartment pressures. 3. **P**allor; decreased capillary perfusion 4. **P**aresthesia. Loss of sensory function is first symptom of a developing compartment syndrome. 5. **P**aralysis 6. **P**ressure; i.e., high measured compartment pressure
Diagnosis?	Measurement of compartment pressures and clinical exam. Important to evaluate compartment pressure in relation to the diastolic blood pressure. Compartment pressures within 30 mm Hg of diastolic blood pressure or greater than 30–40 mm Hg are suggestive of possible syndrome.
Treatment?	Fasciotomy. This is often done prophylactically if the risk of developing a compartment syndrome is high.

FAT EMBOLISM SYNDROME

What is fat embolism syndrome?	Embolization of fat particles from bone marrow
Most common cause?	Long bone fractures
Time of presentation?	Usually within 24–72 hours after fracture
Risk factors?	1. Multiple long bone fractures 2. Delayed fracture immobilization 3. Delayed operative stabilization.

Signs/symptoms?	1. Petechiae (especially in upper trunk and arms), irritability/confusion, tachycardia, and hypoxia 2. Intravascular fat or fat in the urine (rare)
Chest x-ray?	Fluffy infiltrate and interstitial/alveolar pattern resembling adult respiratory distress syndrome (ARDS). Often lags behind clinical picture.
EKG?	Large embolism can cause a right ventricle strain pattern (as in a pulmonary thromboembolism).
Management?	1. Immobilize long bone fracture. 2. Provide supportive care; monitor arterial blood gases (ABG). 3. Ventilatory support should be provided, if needed.

CRUSH SYNDROME

What is crush syndrome?	Renal failure associated with compression injuries to the extremities
Causes?	Combined effects of myoglobin precipitation in renal tubules, hypoxia, hypotension, hyperkalemia, and circulating cytokines
Risk factors?	Prolonged compression/crush of extremity
Signs/symptoms?	Patient appears pale, hypotensive, and hypovolemic
Appearance of urine?	Red to blackish-brown due to myoglobin
Management?	1. Monitor for cardiac effects of hyperkalemia that can kill these patients. 2. Release crushed extremity's compartments early. 3. Replace fluids, treat hyperkalemia. 4. Resect necrotic tissue. 5. Use mannitol to keep urine output high. 6. Alkalinize urine to keep myoglobin soluble.

Complications?	1. Compartment syndrome
	2. Extremity infection/sepsis (necrotic tissue)
	3. Potential lethal arrhythmias, secondary to elevated potassium released from crushed tissue
	4. Systemic inflammatory response syndrome and multisystem organ failure (if soft tissue injury is extensive)

GAS GANGRENE AND CLOSTRIDIUM MYONECROSIS

What is the cause?	90% of cases due to puncture injury and inoculation with *Clostridium perfringens*, an anaerobic, spore-forming, gram-positive rod commonly found in soil, on dirty objects, and in the GI tract.
How often will you see this in your career?	Probably at least once, and it will most likely be disastrous for the patient.
How do you lessen the chance of this disaster?	By checking wounds frequently, especially those that could be contaminated. This possibility is the reason that dressings must be removed and wounds inspected in the febrile postoperative or injured patient.
Signs/symptoms?	Pain out of proportion to what is expected from injury. Swelling/edema, fever, tachycardia, mental status changes, and crepitus are often present.
Characteristic skin color?	Bronze, copper tone. Thin, brown fluid may ooze from injury sites.
Time course?	Early and fast. Signs and symptoms appear within 24–72 hours after injury.
Diagnosis?	History and physical, Gram's stain, CBC with increased WBC count. Must look at all surgical wounds (especially painful ones), even if the operation was very recent.
X-ray?	Air in tissue

Role of culture results?	Minimal in the early phase. Do not wait for culture results to begin treatment.
Treatment?	1. Debridement of necrotic tissue, fasciotomy, or fasciectomy 2. Antibiotics: IV penicillin. If allergic, IV chloramphenicol (aplastic anemia never reported after IV chloramphenicol) 3. Hyperbaric oxygen (controversial) 4. Tetanus prophylaxis

NECROTIZING FASCIITIS

What is the cause?	Most commonly results from inoculation of a dirty traumatic wound, after colonic surgery, or following complications of colonic disease (e.g., perforated diverticulosis)
Most common etiologic agents?	Anaerobic β-hemolytic Streptococcus is most common, but there is almost always a mixed infection with enteric gram-negative organisms and anaerobes (sometimes called "synergistic gangrene").
Signs/symptoms?	Appearance of occasional small-wound infection at skin layer that communicates with fascial layers, hypotension, tachycardia, increased WBC count, unusual amount of pain, fever, tenderness.
Risk factors?	Open fractures, peripheral vascular disease, diabetes—any time there is compromised perfusion, thus favoring an anaerobic environment
Diagnosis?	History and physical (requires a high degree of suspicion, as there may be minimal skin changes early on), Gram stain, CBC with increased WBC count, culture, and sensitivity.
Treatment?	1. Debridement of necrotic tissue often reveals extensive involvement of fascia requiring wide excision 2. Antibiotics for gram-positive, gram-negative, and anaerobic bacteria.

Complications?	Amputation, septic shock, need for skin grafting

NEUROLOGIC TRAUMA

What is the GCS?	Glasgow Coma Scale—an objective assessment of neurologic function and impairment after head injury. A score of 15 is normal; 13 or less is indicative of significant head injury.

How is the GCS calculated?	Eye opening (E)
	  4 = Opens spontaneously
	  3 = Opens to voice (command)
	  2 = Opens to painful stimulus
	  1 = Does not open eyes
	Motor response (M)
	  6 = Obeys commands
	  5 = Localizes painful stimulus
	  4 = Withdraws from pain
	  3 = Decorticate posture
	  2 = Decerebrate posture
	  1 = No movement
	Verbal response (V)
	  5 = Appropriate and oriented
	  4 = Confused
	  3 = Inappropriate words
	  2 = Incomprehensible sounds
	  1 = No sounds

What are the indications for intracranial pressure monitoring following head trauma?	A GCS of less than 9 or the requirement for operative evacuation of traumatic mass lesion.
What is ICP?	Intracranial pressure.
What is CPP?	Cerebral perfusion pressure (CPP = mean arterial pressure [MAP]– intracranial pressure [ICP])
How can you treat a sudden increase in ICP?	1. Elevate head of bed 2. Hyperventilate to decrease PCO_2 (about 30 mm Hg) 3. Mannitol infusion 4. Sedation and paralysis 5. Craniectomy

What complications most frequently cause a sudden neurologic deficit in the ICU trauma patient?	Intracranial hematoma (epidural/subdural), cerebral edema, delayed intracerebral hemorrhage

THORACIC TRAUMA

What is the significance of severe chest wall trauma?	Potential for underlying lung injury
What is the significance of first or second rib fractures?	Very little specific significance. These findings do indicate that enough energy transfer occurred to possibly cause intrathoracic injury, such as aortic disruption. However, mediastinal widening is the most sensitive indicator of aortic injury.
What are the indications for thoracotomy after chest tube placement in a patient with chest trauma?	An initial output from the chest tube of 1,500–2,000 ml, or more than 150–200 ml/hr for more than 2–4 hours.
What are the major issues in treating patients with pulmonary contusions?	Avoid overhydration and volume overload, and maintain optimal pulmonary toilet. These patients may need ventilatory support.
Why is it important to thoroughly drain a traumatic hemothorax?	Complications of undrained hemothorax include fibrothorax, with subsequent loss of lung volume, and empyema (infection of the residual blood).
What are other terms for ARDS?	1. Noncardiogenic pulmonary edema 2. Shock lung
What causes the greatest morbidity from flail chest?	The underlying pulmonary contusion.
What is the most effective treatment for pulmonary contusion and rib fractures in the awake, cooperative patient?	A vigorous pulmonary toilet. Intubation should be avoided if possible. Rib blocks are not very helpful because they must be repeated every 6–8 hours. Epidural anesthesia can be considered.

When should chest tubes be left in the trauma patient?

1. Total drainage of more than 100 ml in 24 hours
2. Recurrence of pneumothorax on water seal
3. Patient still on positive pressure ventilation
4. If any doubt about the need for tube exists. Leaving chest tubes in never causes problems. Removing them prematurely can be deadly.

23

Burn Patients

What are some statistics regarding burns in the United States?

1. Overall incidence is 2 million annually; 3%–5% are life-threatening.
2. Approximately 100,000 burn patients require hospital care.
3. Approximately 20,000 fatalities occur as a result of the injury or its complications.
4. Burns are the second leading cause of death in individuals from birth to 12 years of age.

What is the largest organ of the body?

The skin

What is involved in the initial evaluation of a burn victim?

Remember the **ABC**s:
Airway
Breathing
Circulation

What is the first treatment step for any burn?

1. Stop the burning process.
2. Immediately remove all clothes.
3. Remove hot and adherent substances such as grease and tar.
4. Copiously irrigate all chemical burns with water.
5. Chemical eye burns require prolonged (up to 8 hours) flushing.

What is the most common error in the care of burn patients?

Delay in treatment. Many complications of severe burns, including renal failure and sepsis, are severely aggravated by inadequate or delayed fluid resuscitation.

What are the hospitalization criteria for burn patients?

1. Second-degree burns greater than 20% total body surface area (TBSA)
2. Third-degree burns greater than 10% TBSA
3. Any burns greater than 10% TBSA in children and the elderly
4. Any burns involving the face, hands, feet, or perineum

5. Any burns with inhalation injury
6. Any burns with associated trauma
7. Any electrical burns

Why is it important to monitor temperature closely in the burn patient?

Temperature tends to be very labile due to exposure, fluid losses with evaporation, administration of large volumes of hypothermic fluids, and central temperature instability. Hypothermia predisposes to cardiac irritability and coagulopathy.

How are minor burns dressed?

Minor burns are treated initially with cold compresses for pain relief. After gentle cleaning with nonionic detergent and debridement of loose skin and broken blisters, the burn is dressed with a topical antibacterial (silver sulfadiazine, neomycin) and covered with a sterile dressing.

How are major burns dressed?

After gentle cleaning only, the burns are dressed with topical antibiotic and sterile dressings; cold compresses are avoided. Gentle debridement through dressing changes and over several days allows second-degree burns to heal and prepares third-degree burns for grafting.

Note some advantages and disadvantages of each antibacterial agent.

1. Silver nitrate—broad spectrum, painless and inexpensive, but nonpenetrating and may cause electrolyte imbalance
2. Silver sulfadiazine (Silvadene)— painless, no electrolyte imbalances, no need for occlusive dressing, little penetration, misses *Pseudomonas*, and has idiosyncratic neutropenia; agent of choice for small burns.
3. Mafenide (sulfamylon)—penetrates eschars, broad spectrum (but misses *Staphylococcus*), but pain and burning on application; allergic reaction in 7%; may cause acid-base imbalances (carbonic anhydrase inhibition); agent of choice in already-contaminated burn wounds.

What is important medical history, even in the case of a minor burn?

Tetanus status, allergies to neomycin or sulfa

How many layers comprise the epidermis?

Five

Which layer plays a major role in H₂O retention?

The stratum corneum

What is the significance of burns that obliterate the stratum corneum?

Results in increased evaporative losses of water

Where do the blood vessels responsible for heat regulation lie?

The dermis

Name the zones that are associated with local burn injury.

1. Zone of coagulation: nonviable, no blood flow
2. Zone of stasis: microvascular sludging
3. Zone of hyperemia: viable tissue

What are the degrees of severity used to describe burn wounds?

First, second, and third. First- and second-degree = partial thickness; third-degree = full thickness

Can infection convert a partial thickness into a full thickness injury?

Yes!

What are the characteristics of a first-degree burn?

1. The epidermis only is involved.
2. Blistering does not occur (looks like a bad sunburn), and little if any tissue death occurs.
3. Skin is painful, pink, and dry with slight edema and brisk capillary refill.

What are the characteristics of a second-degree burn?

1. Injury involves the epidermis and dermis and some portions of the hair follicles, sweat glands, and stratum germinatum.
2. Injured tissue still blanches and sensation remains intact.
3. Burn can be superficial or deep, and blistering occurs.
4. This type of burn is also defined as a partial-thickness burn.

What are the characteristics of a third-degree burn?

1. Full thickness (all layers of skin are affected)
2. Loss of sensation/insensitive to pain
3. Thrombosis of blood vessels
4. Appears white, red, or black, with marked edema
5. Requires skin grafting

What are the characteristics of a fourth-degree burn?

Burned to the muscle or bone. Requires extensive flaps, grafting, or amputation.

Is debridement of blisters indicated?

No, they provide protection of underlying tissue.

Burn severity is determined by which measure?

The TBSA affected by second- and third-degree burns; TBSA is calculated by the "rule of nines" in adults and by a modified rule in children to account for the disproportionate size of the head and trunk.

What is "burn shock?"

Hypovolemic shock secondary to massive fluid shifts into the injured area and interstitial space.

Most critical areas for burns?

Face, ears, hands, over joints, and perineum

What is the best method to monitor adequacy of fluid resuscitation?

Urinary output via a Foley catheter. Urine output should be maintained at greater than 1/2 ml/kg/hr in adults and at greater than 1 ml/kg/hr in children. If urine output is unreliable (renal or heart failure), use a pulmonary artery catheter.

What type of IV fluid should be used in the initial resuscitation and in the initial 24 hours after burn injury?

Lactated Ringer's solution

When is it appropriate to use colloid as a volume expander?

After the first 24 hours, i.e., once leaking injured capillaries begin to seal

What is the Parkland formula?

1. It calculates the volume of lactated Ringer's solution needed for resuscitation in the first 24 hours after injury, based on burn surface area (BSA).
2. Total 24-hour fluid requirement = 4 ml/kg × %BSA involved with second- or third-degree burns
3. Half of the calculated volume is given over the first 8 hours, and the other half over the ensuing 16 hours.

How is the crystalloid given?

Through two large-bore peripheral venous catheters introduced through unburned skin.

Does this formula work in children?

No. Use 6 ml × weight (kg) × %total BSA.

What factors warrant an increase in fluid requirements?

Inhalation injury, delay in resuscitation, escharotomies, electrical injuries, alcohol/drugs, use of mannitol for myoglobinuria.

What is the "rule of nines?"

Method used to estimate BSA. The body is divided into eleven areas, each comprising approximately 9% (head 9%, arms 9% each, legs 18% each, back 18%, front 18%, perineum 1%). The formula is not accurate in small children in whom the head comprises a larger BSA and the legs a lower BSA.

What is the quickest way to estimate the burn area?

The palm equals about 1% BSA.

Are prophylactic antibiotics indicated in severe burn injuries?

No. They do not decrease the incidence of burn wound sepsis but do select for resistant organisms.

Should tetanus prophylaxis be given to all burn victims?

Yes, except those patients actively immunized within the preceding 12 months

What is an eschar?

Carbonization of tissue caused by heat

Circumferential, full-thickness burns to the extremities are at risk for what complication?	Distal neurovascular impairment, which is similar to compartment syndrome
How is it treated?	Escharotomy, which is a full-thickness longitudinal incision through the eschar with scalpel or electrocautery; incision must extend into healthy fat.
What are the indications for performance of an escharotomy in a burned extremity?	1. Decreased pulses or decreased capillary refill 2. Change in neurologic exam, i.e., developing paresthesia or loss of sensory or motor function 3. Peripheral cyanosis. (An O_2-saturation monitor may be placed on an extremity to monitor this. It will not read if blood flow is compromised.)
Why should an escharotomy of the chest wall be done?	To prevent impediment of respiratory excursions and resultant loss of tidal volume
What are the effects of major burns on the GI tract?	1. Adynamic ileus and gastric dilatation. (Be sure to place a nasogastric tube to low constant suction in all patients with burns greater than 20% BSA.) 2. Curling's ulcer
What is a Curling's ulcer?	Gastric ulcer that develops in burn patients secondary to loss of cytoprotective effects of gastric mucus and increased acid secretion.
How is a Curling's ulcer prevented?	H_2 blockers, carafate, and/or antacids. Keep gastric pH above 4. Provide early enteral feedings (within 24 hours).

INHALATION INJURIES

What is the incidence of inhalation injuries?	10%–20% of hospitalized burn patients

Symptoms suggestive of inhalation injury?

Singed nasal hairs, circumoral or intraoral burns, hoarseness, rasping cough or altered phonation, hemoptysis, wheezing, history of confinement in a closed space, hypoxia, bronchoscopic evidence of airway edema, inflammation, mucosal necrosis, and carbon deposits. Need for prolonged ventilatory support may also be suggestive of lower airway damage from an inhalation injury.

What is the best way to confirm upper airway inhalation injury?

Direct laryngoscopy with fiberoptic bronchoscope

What is the associated mortality of burn patients with inhalation injuries?

40%–50%, as compared to approximately 10% for patients without inhalation injuries. (The presence of an inhalation injury is a major determinant of mortality.)

What area of the respiratory tract is most susceptible to direct thermal injury?

Upper airways, especially the epiglottis

Where does smoke inhalation cause most injury?

Bronchial tree and alveolar membranes

What is a common cause of upper airway obstruction?

Edema of the laryngeal structures

What is the best treatment of upper airway injury?

Endotracheal intubation

How does smoke inhalation injure the respiratory tree?

1. Epithelial disruption
2. Decreases mucociliary clearance
3. Incites an inflammatory response with increased blood flow and airway edema formation
4. Increases permeability of the alveolar-capillary membrane with subsequent interstitial edema and alveolar flooding

What other gaseous substances accompany smoke inhalation and are a source of morbidity?	Cyanide and carbon monoxide (CO)
How does CO interfere with oxygen delivery?	Reversibly displaces O_2 from the hemoglobin molecule forming carboxyhemoglobin. Carboxyhemoglobin interferes with the mitochondrial cytochrome oxidase-a3 complex, thereby decreasing O_2 utilization as well.
What is the affinity of CO to Hgb compared to O_2?	200 times greater
How long does it take to eliminate CO (i.e., what is the T1/2 of elimination)?	250 minutes while breathing room air. Note that it drops to 40–60 minutes if inspiring 100% O_2 or 30 minutes in hyperbaric O_2 chamber.
What is a normal CO level?	10% in smokers and 5% in nonsmokers
What are some signs of CO poisoning?	Headache, nausea, vomiting, lethargy, mental status changes
What is the Rx for CO poisoning?	1. 100% supplemental O_2 2. Intubation if mental status changes occur 3. Hyperbaric oxygen (2 atmospheres) if available
What is the mechanism of cyanide poisoning?	Disrupts oxidative phosphorylation by binding to cytochrome-a3 complex, resulting in lactic acidosis and cell death
Cyanide toxicity comes from what?	Burning plastic and polyurethane
What are the signs of cyanide poisoning?	1. Persistent metabolic acidosis despite adequate fluid resuscitation 2. Increased venous O_2 content (impaired O_2 utilization)
What is the treatment for cyanide poisoning?	Amylnitrite, sodium nitrite, sodium thiosulphate, and vitamin B_{12}

Is the administration of steroids indicated to reduce airway swelling in the setting of inhalation injuries?

NO, as this probably also increases the risk of infection.

What is the Rx for suspected upper airway injury?

Orotracheal intubation to prevent acute upper airway occlusion secondary to edema formation

What maneuvers can be used to decrease upper airway edema?

Elevate the head of patient's bed to 30 degrees.

In an intubated patient, how can the resolution of airway edema be assessed?

Deflation of the endotracheal tube cuff will allow audible passage of air around the tube if airway swelling has resolved to the point where extubation can be considered.

What other signs are useful to help judge the resolution of airway edema?

Decreased facial and periorbital edema. Note that direct laryngoscopy is helpful in assessing the supraglottic region.

In a burn patient with an inhalation injury, should fluid resuscitation be minimized to avoid pulmonary edema?

No, adequate fluid resuscitation is necessary to maintain cardiopulmonary stability. In fact, patients with an inhalation injury may require an even greater volume of fluids than an isolated burn injury.

What are some of the sequelae of inhalation injuries?

Increased incidence of nosocomial pneumonia and adult respiratory distress syndrome (ARDS). Serious long-term sequelae are rare, however.

ELECTRICAL INJURIES

What is the incidence of electrical injury?

Approximately 1% of all accidental deaths. (Note that 25% of these are due to lightning.)

What are the two major types of electrical burn injuries?

1. Electrical arc injuries where the current passes external to the body, causing local burns at the sites of contact
2. Injuries where the current passes through the body

What factors determine the magnitude of injury?	1. Type of current 2. Amount of current 3. Pathway of current 4. Duration of contact 5. Area of contact 6. Resistance of the body 7. Voltage
Which layer of the skin is responsible for most resistance to electrical current?	Stratum corneum, which acts as an insulator of deeper tissues. (Note that surface resistance drops dramatically if wet.)
Why are electric burns so dangerous?	Most of the destruction from electrical burns is internal, as the route of least electrical resistance follows nerves, blood vessels, and fascia. Injury is usually far worse than external burns at entrance and exit sites would indicate. Cardiac arrhythmias, myoglobinuria, acidosis, and renal failure are common.
What is Ohm's law and what is its significance?	Current = voltage/resistance. (Current is directly responsible for injury; therefore, the higher the voltage and the lower the resistance, the greater the current and resultant injury.)
What is AC?	Alternating current. Electron flow reverses at a given frequency; note that this is the usual form of commercial current.
What is "let-go" current?	Amount of current above which involuntary muscle contractions prevent victim from escaping current's source (approximately 15 milliamperes [mA]).
What effect does electric current have on the respiratory system?	If the amount of current exceeds approximately 20 mA, it can cause tetany of the respiratory muscles and result in asphyxia if the source of the current is not removed.
What are some considerations in management of electrical burns?	Cardiac monitoring, cardiac enzymes, treatment of myoglobinuria

What effect does electric current have on the cardiac system?	If the current exceeds 30–40 mA, ventricular fibrillation may be induced. Current is dependent on the duration of shock and weight of the individual. However, at very high currents, complete depolarization occurs; once the source is removed, the heart will convert to normal sinus rhythm (i.e., defibrillation).
What is the Rx for a low-voltage burn victim who is without vital signs once removed from the source of the current?	Initiation of CPR and ACLS protocols
What determines the path of a high-voltage electrical current passing through the body?	The current will follow the shortest path between contact points and involve the structures in its path.
What is the significance of entrance and exit wounds?	They signify local destruction to deeper tissues, which is often grossly underestimated.
What is the significance of underlying muscle tissue injury?	Tissue damage with extravasation of fluid and subsequent swelling may result in fascial compartment syndromes.
What are the symptoms and signs of a developing compartment syndrome?	The **five Ps:** 1. **P**ain 2. **P**aresthesias 3. **P**allor 4. **P**aralysis 5. **P**ulselessness
What other complications can significant muscle necrosis cause?	Renal failure and hyperkalemia secondary to rhabdomyolysis
What is rhabdomyolysis?	Injury to muscle causing myoglobin in the urine; often seen in electrical or crush injuries
How is the diagnosis of rhabdomyolysis made?	1. Presence of dark, tea-colored urine 2. Urine positive for myoglobin and other hemochromogens (dipstick positive for blood but no RBCs on microscopic examination)

3. Elevated creatine phosphokinase (CPK) in blood

What is the Rx for myoglobinuria?

1. Maintain urine output greater than 100 ml/hr with vigorous IV fluids and mannitol.
2. Alkalinize urine with IV bicarbonate to prevent precipitation of myoglobin in renal tubules.

What are the common GI complications of electrical injuries?

1. Adynamic ileus
2. Stress ulcers (Curling's ulcers)

MALIGNANT HYPERTHERMIA

What is malignant hyperthermia?

A metabolic defect resulting in uncontrolled muscle contraction and the uncoupling of oxidative phosphorylation.

How is it inherited?

Autosomal dominant inheritance with variable penetrance

How is the reaction set off?

Exposure to inhalation anesthetic agents (i.e., halothane, enflurane, etc.); also can be triggered with exposure to succinylcholine

What are the early signs?

Increased temperature, tachypnea, tachycardia, cyanosis, rigidity, increased CO_2 production, diaphoresis, labile blood pressure, and failure of muscle relaxation with adequate doses of succinylcholine

What are the late findings?

Lactic acidosis, respiratory acidosis (from increased CO_2 production), hyperkalemia, increased serum CK levels, myoglobinemia, myoglobinuria

What is the mechanism?

Believed to be due to altered calcium homeostasis within muscle tissue that leads to high intracellular Ca^{++} and activation of phosphorylase kinase. This ultimately leads to uncontrolled muscle contraction, uncoupling of phosphorylation, and excessive production of heat, CO_2, and lactate.

What is the Rx?	1. Hydration, body cooling, intubation, and hyperventilation
	2. Sodium bicarbonate and diuretics to maintain urine output
	3. Dantrolene sodium, which blocks excitation-contraction coupling between the T-tubules and the SR. (The dose is 1–2 mg/kg, which can be repeated at 5-minute intervals for a total of 10 mg/kg.)
Is a family history helpful?	Yes. Preoperative questioning concerning family history of anesthetic problems may alter anesthetic techniques used.

MALIGNANT NEUROLEPTIC SYNDROME

What is malignant neuroleptic syndrome?	Syndrome of hyperthermia, autonomic instability, increased muscle rigidity, and myoglobinuria in susceptible patients exposed to neuroleptics
What is the incidence?	Occurs in fewer than 1% of patients exposed to neuroleptics
What is the time course of the developing syndrome?	The syndrome evolves over 1–3 days after initiation of neuroleptic treatment and will continue for approximately 1 week after the neuroleptic has been discontinued.
What is the Rx?	1. Discontinue the offending agent.
	2. As in malignant hyperthermia, dantrolene is the agent of choice.
	3. Supportive care
What is the associated mortality?	Approximately 25%

FROSTBITE

What factors predispose to frostbite injuries?	Alcoholism and psychiatric illness

What are the mechanisms of injury?

1. Cellular dehydration
2. Ice crystal formation within the tissue (both intracellular and extracellular)
3. Microvascular occlusion

How is the vasculature affected?

1. Upon thawing, increased permeability occurs, with subsequent plasma fluid leaking into the interstitium
2. Hemoconcentration in the microvascular beds results in platelet aggregation and thrombosis.

What is the "Hunting reaction?"

Alternating peripheral vasodilatation and vasoconstriction that occurs when extremity temperatures decrease to below 10°C. The response is an effort to slow the freezing process; however, preservation of core temperature is sacrificed.

How are frostbite injuries classified?

By the appearance of the extremity after thawing.
First degree: hyperemia, edema, superficial freezing of the epidermis
Second degree: hyperemia, edema, vesicle formation (cutaneous sensation remains intact)
Third degree: Necrosis of all skin layers extending into subcutaneous tissues
Fourth degree: Full thickness injury that extends into the underlying bone and muscle

Is motor function always impaired in severe injuries?

NO. Proximal muscles and tendons may remain intact, allowing movement of distal extremities.

What is the Rx for frostbite injuries?

1. Rapid rewarming in 40°C water bath
2. Narcotics to relieve pain
3. Leave vesicles intact as they protect underlying tissue
4. Daily wound care and whirlpool therapy
5. Avoidance of further trauma to the injured extremity (i.e., bed rest, foot cradles, sheepskins, etc.)
6. Surgical intervention/debridement, but this must be delayed until

demarcation is clear and may take several weeks. Early estimates of tissue damage often overestimate the extent of nonviable tissue. Note, however, that progression to wet gangrene requires early debridement.

Is rapid rewarming of the extremity indicated?

YES, as it provides a chance for marginal tissues to recover. Immersion in a 40°C water bath with adequate circulation is optimal.

Are fasciotomies indicated in severe injuries?

NO, because vessels are already thrombosed rather than merely constricted by tissue swelling.

HYPOTHERMIA

What is the hallmark of hypothermia?

Core body temperature below 34°C.

What is the most common symptom?

Altered mental status

What are some other signs?

Decreased heart rate, blood pressure, and respiratory rate

What is the most important therapeutic intervention?

Rapid initiation of rewarming

What is the Rx?

Warm IV fluids and "passive" rewarming (warm blankets, warming lights, increase room temperature, etc.) if core temperature is above 28°C and patient is shivering.

When is "active" rewarming indicated?

1. Asystole
2. Core temperature below 28°C
3. Failure of passive rewarming.

What are the methods of active rewarming?

1. Total body immersion in 40°C water bath
2. Warm lavage via chest tube thoracostomy
3. Cardiopulmonary bypass

What monitoring is essential during rewarming?

1. EKG (for development of arrhythmias, most of which are supraventricular)
2. Monitoring of electrolytes (tendency toward hypokalemia)

24

Transplant Patients

DEFINITIONS

Autograft?	Same individual is donor and recipient.
Isograft?	Donor and recipient are genetically identical (identical twins).
Allograft?	Donor and recipient are genetically dissimilar but of the same species.
Xenograft?	Donor and recipient belong to different species.
Orthotopic?	Donor organ is placed in anatomic position (liver, heart).
Heterotopic?	Donor organ is placed in different anatomic position (kidney, pancreas).
Paratopic?	Donor organ is placed close to original organ.

TRANSPLANT INFECTION

What two groups of infections are more common in transplant patients than in other ICU patients?	Fungi and viruses
When are infections most common after any transplant?	During the first 3–6 months
What type of infections are most common after transplantation (other than a "cold")?	Bacterial (common), atypical bacterial, followed by viral, fungal, and protozoal

What process can masquerade with fever and an infiltrate following organ transplantation?	Transplant-associated B-cell lymphoma, which occurs in 1%–5% of patients over time. (The frequency depends on the organ transplanted.)
When is prophylactic amphotericin B indicated in the transplant patient?	After re-explorations or retransplants, secondary to the high incidence of postoperative fungal infections
What is the most common cause of viral pneumonia in transplant patients?	Cytomegalovirus (CMV)
What is the treatment of choice for CMV?	Ganciclovir
What is the most common complication of ganciclovir?	Leukopenia
What antiviral agent can be used if ganciclovir toxicity (usually bone marrow suppression) occurs?	Foscarnet (acyclovir can also be used)
What organ systems are most frequently involved with CMV?	• GI (stomach, colon) • Lung (pneumonitis) • Other (heart, etc.). CMV infections can also stimulate the immune system and, therefore, are frequently associated with rejection.
What fungus is usually fatal in transplant patients if isolated from the brain?	*Aspergillus*
What virus most commonly causes encephalitis in transplant patients?	Herpes simplex virus (HSV)
What is the treatment of choice for HSV infection?	High-dose IV acyclovir
Why is Bactrim used in transplant patients?	For prophylaxis against *Pneumocystis carinii*

What four organisms cause nonspecific pulmonary infiltrates in transplant patients?	*Legionella, Aspergillus, Histoplasma,* and *Cryptococcus*
What is the test of choice to evaluate serious infiltrates?	Bronchoalveolar lavage
What foreign body is a common cause of sepsis in the liver transplant patients?	IV catheters

IMMUNOSUPPRESSION

Who needs to be immunosuppressed?	All recipients (except auto- or isograft recipients)
How do the following immunosuppressive agents work?	
Azathioprine (AZT)?	Blocks mitosis and proliferation of competent lymphoid cells and inhibits synthesis and function of both DNA and RNA.
Corticosteroids?	Inhibit production of interleukin (IL)-1 from macrophages
Cyclosporine (CSA)?	Inhibits IL-2 release from activated T-helper cells
Antilymphocyte drugs?	1. Monoclonal OKT-3: blocks CD-3 receptors on T cells, thus preventing antigen recognition. 2. Polyclonal antithymocyte γ-globulin/ antilymphocyte globulin (ATGAM/ ALG): fixes complement and lyses T lymphocytes.
What is three-drug therapy?	Cyclosporine, azathioprine, prednisone
What medications lower cyclosporine levels?	• Dilantin • Phenobarbital • Rifampin • Isoniazid

What medications raise cyclosporine levels?	• Macrolides (e.g., erythromycin) • Ketoconazole, itraconazole • Diltiazem • Amiodarone
What medications may potentiate renal dysfunction when used with cyclosporine?	• Aminoglycosides • Amphotericin • Nonsteroidal anti-inflammatory agents
Name six side effects of steroids?	1. Glucose intolerance 2. Adrenal insufficiency if acutely withdrawn 3. Cataracts 4. Osteoporosis 5. Cushingoid appearance 6. Skin fragility
When is rejection most common (any organ)?	Within the first 1–2 months
What two drugs are used to treat acute organ rejection?	Glucocorticoids and OKT-3 (for steroid-resistant rejection)
What is the most common life-threatening complication of OKT-3 therapy?	Severe pulmonary edema
What are the most common side effects of the following agents, requiring dose or agent change? **AZT**	Leukopenia, thrombocytopenia, pancreatitis
CSA	Nephrotoxicity, hypertension, tremulousness
Antithymocyte globulin (ATG)	Thrombocytopenia/leukopenia. May cause anaphylaxis or pulmonary edema.
OKT-3	Pulmonary edema

KIDNEY TRANSPLANT

What are the two major causes of immediate nonfunction of a cadaveric renal transplant?

1. Hyperacute rejection
2. Technical problem with anastomosis

Does cold ischemic time affect the degree of acute tubular necrosis (ATN) in a cadaveric renal transplant?

Yes. The longer the time of cold ischemia, the greater the degree of ATN may be. Living related donors have less ATN because of lack of cold ischemic time.

What is the best measure of postoperative renal function?

Urine output (UOP). Blood urea nitrogen (BUN) and creatinine may also be helpful.

What central venous pressure (CVP) is generally maintained in a postoperative renal transplant?

12–15 mm Hg

How can one estimate the IV fluid needed to maintain adequate CVP in a transplant patient?

Input = output + 50 ml/hr in adults

If CVP is adequate and UOP is low, what is the next management, diuretics or vasopressors?

Diuretics: Lasix (100–200 mg IV); Bumex (3–5 mg IV); metolazone (10–30 mg IV)

Why should vasopressors be avoided?

Vasospasm and decreased renal perfusion may lead to vascular thrombosis and loss of graft.

Why are fluids given to the postoperative kidney transplant patient, even with a good urine output (> 30 ml/hr), to keep CVP above or equal to 10?

1. The denervated transplant kidney is solely dependent on pressure for perfusion.
2. Intraoperative diuretics (mannitol and Lasix) may cause spuriously high urine output.

What radiographic test should be obtained if the kidney does not have adequate UOP despite adequate CVP and diuretics?

Doppler ultrasound to assess vascular flow

If the Doppler confirms adequate flow and there is still no UOP, what is the next step?

Hemodialysis

How can you differentiate ATN from rejection?

Transplant kidney biopsy

What immunosuppressive agents are used in the immediate postoperative cadaveric transplant recipient?

OKT-3, AZT, corticosteroids, ATGAM (antilymphocyte preparations)

Why is CSA not generally used in the first 3 days after cadaveric renal transplant?

CSA causes arteriolar vasoconstriction especially in the kidney. This may accentuate vasospasm, ATN, and poor graft function.

If a renal biopsy is done and shows acute cellular rejection, what treatment is initiated?

Corticosteroid bolus with taper

If the kidney fails to respond to steroids, what is the next step?

OKT-3

What is a life-threatening complication of OKT-3 therapy?

Pulmonary edema

What clinical and laboratory signs are suggestive of a urine leak?

Clear fluid leakage from the wound and an increase in serum creatinine

How can a urine leak be diagnosed?

1. Send wound fluid for BUN and creatinine
2. Ultrasound can show fluid collections or outlet obstruction
3. Mag 3 scan for perfusion and excretion

PANCREAS TRANSPLANT

What parameters are followed in pancreas transplant recipients?	Urinary amylase, blood glucose (also, parameters for kidney transplant if the recipient is having a combined pancreas/kidney transplant)
What vessels provide the blood supply to the transplanted pancreas the majority of the time?	The iliac artery and the iliac vein
How is the exocrine pancreas drained?	Via a duodenal segment anastomosed to the bladder
What should you do if UOP is zero and clots are seen in the Foley bag?	Irrigate the Foley every hour to avoid ongoing obstruction as this may cause bladder distension and lead to an anastomotic leak.
What CVP should be maintained for a pancreas transplant patient?	12–15 mm Hg, the same as for a cadaveric renal transplant patient.
What fluid rate should be maintained?	Input = output + 50 ml/hr when CVP is greater than 10. If CVP is greater than 18, decrease to input = output.
Is glucose placed in the maintenance fluid in the immediate postoperative period?	No
How is glucose managed in the immediate postoperative period?	A separate infusion of D10W at 20 ml/hr should be infused with an insulin drip initiated at 1 U/hr and titrate each to maintain glucose level of 80–150 mg/dl.
What is the most common cause of early graft loss?	Thrombosis
What additional agent can be infused to attempt to prevent graft thrombosis?	Low–molecular-weight dextran at 20 ml/hr
What laboratory studies are suggestive of rejection in a pancreas transplant?	Decreased urinary amylase in units/hr (to avoid urine volume variation) and increased blood glucose

How is the diagnosis of pancreatic rejection made?	Biopsy of the associated kidney. If no kidney was transplanted with the pancreas, rejection is the presumptive diagnosis based on the blood glucose and urinary amylase. The transplanted pancreas is not biopsied.
Which organ usually rejects first in the combined procedure, the kidney or the pancreas?	Usually the kidney
Is there better long-term graft survival with pancreas transplant alone or with combined pancreas-kidney transplantation?	Combined pancreas-kidney transplantation
Would fluid requirements tend to be higher for a cadaver renal transplant or for a combined pancreas-kidney transplant?	A pancreas-kidney transplant is generally done through an open abdominal procedure and has much higher third-space losses.

LIVER TRANSPLANT

What four parameters are used to assess intravascular volume in a postoperative liver transplant patient?	CVP, pulmonary artery diastolic (PAD) pressure, pulmonary capillary wedge pressure (PCWP), UOP
What is the primary clinical measure of adequate perfusion?	UOP
What UOP is the lowest acceptable output in the adult and child?	Adult: 0.5 ml/kg/hr; child: 1–2 ml/kg/hr
What unusual fluid loss is replaced in an immediate postoperative liver transplant patient?	The fluid from three Jackson-Pratt drains is replaced ml for ml with 5% albumin for the first 48 hours.

At what PT value after transplantation is fresh frozen plasma (FFP) transfused in the early postoperative period?	PT greater than 25 or if the patient is clinically bleeding; otherwise, correction at lower values may interfere with assessment of synthetic function of the new liver.
What is primary nonfunction?	Unexplained factors that cause the transplanted liver to not function, requiring emergent retransplantation.
When is CSA started as immunosuppressive therapy for liver?	Intraoperatively
What is the most common hematologic disorder seen in postoperative liver transplant patients?	Thrombocytopenia
What is the work-up for increased liver function tests (LFTs), increased PT, and increased bilirubin?	Doppler ultrasound to ensure hepatic arterial flow and intraductal dilation, which are technical problems; a T-tube cholangiogram to evaluate biliary obstruction; finally, a liver biopsy to rule out rejection
What parameters are followed to assess postoperative liver transplant function?	Bile quantity and quality, lactic acid levels, PT/PTT (coagulation studies), ammonia levels
What is the most common indication for early re-exploration of liver transplant patients?	Bleeding
What is the main indication for later re-exploration?	Sepsis

CARDIAC TRANSPLANT

How is acute rejection in a cardiac transplant diagnosed?	Endomyocardial biopsy

What medication should not be used to treat bradycardia following heart transplantation?	Atropine
What medications should be used to treat bradycardia following heart transplantation?	Epinephrine, isoproterenol
What medication should not be used to treat supraventricular tachycardias following heart transplantation?	Digoxin; the long-term use of β-blockers is also generally discouraged, as these agents reduce exercise tolerance.
Why are tachy-, brady-, dysrhythmias treated differently in heart transplant recipients?	The heart is denervated; therefore, vagolytic (atropine) and vagotonic (digoxin) agents are not effective (as stated previously).
Can a heart transplant patient have a heart attack?	Yes; coronary artery disease (CAD) is a manifestation of chronic rejection. About 50% of heart transplant patients have some evidence of CAD at 5 years; this is usually significant in only 5%.
Does reinnervation ever occur?	Yes; 75% of heart recipients show some sympathetic reinnervation after 1 year.
Does reinnervation have any practical implication?	Yes; patients who reinnervate have improved exercise performance (faster heart rate response); also, some recipients who develop CAD complain of chest pain.
How long can a heart or lung remain ischemic?	Approximately 4 hours (which determines how far you can travel to retrieve organs)
What is the most common arrhythmia?	Bradycardia
What is the treatment for bradycardia?	Chronotropes (Isoprel) and pacing

What factors are important for successful heart, lung, and heart-lung transplantation?

ABO compatibility and approximate size match

In a heart-lung transplant recipient, is it possible to reject a lung without concomitant heart rejection?

Yes; either lung may show evidence of rejection without involvement of the opposite lung or the heart.

LUNG TRANSPLANT

What is the definition of rejection in a lung transplant?

Fever, infiltrate, and hypoxia that responds to antirejection medications

Lung transplantation may be appropriate therapy for selected patients with end-stage pulmonary disease. What are some common indications for lung transplantation?

Chronic obstructive pulmonary disease (COPD), pulmonary fibrosis, cystic fibrosis, α-1 antitrypsin deficiency, and primary pulmonary hypertension are the most common indications for a lung transplant.

Patients with cystic fibrosis receive double lung transplants, whereas patients with COPD commonly receive only single lung transplants. Why is this?

Patients with cystic fibrosis uniformly have chronic bacterial infection in both lungs. If a single lung transplant were done, the patient's nontransplanted lung would serve as a nidus of infection, which is particularly troublesome with the necessary immunosuppression.

A patient has a new infiltrate in the transplanted side on the chest radiograph 10 days after single lung transplantation. What is the differential diagnosis?

The major differential is between infection (pneumonia) and rejection of the graft.

How can you determine if the infiltrate is due to infection?

Bronchoscopy and bronchoalveolar lavage, or BAL. BAL is the irrigation of a segmental bronchus with a small volume of saline. The specimen is analyzed for white cell counts and sent for culture and Gram's stain. High white cell counts in the BAL fluid are suggestive of infection.

How can you determine if the infiltrate is due to rejection?

Bronchoscopy and transbronchial biopsy, or TBB. TBB is performed by passing a small biopsy forceps out through a subsegmental bronchus into the lung parenchyma. The specimens are stained and examined for evidence of a perivascular lymphocytic infiltrate, which is the hallmark of acute cellular rejection. In practice, it is often performed along with a BAL.

When seeing a patient after lung transplantation with dyspnea and a new lung infiltrate, what should you consider?

Rejection, infection

What is the differential diagnosis of lung recipients with dyspnea who wheeze?

- Infection
- Rejection
- Anastomotic stenosis (bronchial)
- Disease of the nontransplanted lung (COPD, asthma, etc.)
- Cardiac disease

What is the differential diagnosis of lung recipients who are hypoxic?

- Infection
- Rejection (acute)
- Bronchiolitis obliterans (chronic rejection)
- Anastomotic stenosis (pulmonary artery)
- Cardiac disease

Index

Page numbers in *italics* represent figures; page numbers with *t* indicate tables.

Titles to Make the Most of Your Clerkship Experience

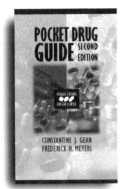

___ Abelow: Understanding Acid-Base
___ Bauer: Mount Sinai Handbook of Surgery
___ Beckmann: Obstetrics and Gynecology
___ Bernstein: Pediatrics
___ Byrne: Publishing Your Medical Research Papers
___ Daffner: Clinical Radiology
___ Gean: Index to Prescription Drugs
___ Gean: Pocket Drug Guide
___ Kutty: Concise Textbook of Medicine
___ Lawrence: Essentials of General Surgery
___ Lawrence: Essentials of Surgical Specialties
___ Rucker: Essentials of Adult Ambulatory Care
___ Sloane: Essentials of Family Medicine
___ Stedman's Medical Dictionary, 26th ed

House Officer Series:
___ Aluisio: Orthopaedics
___ Berry: Anesthesiology
___ Burch: Endocrinology
___ Heger: Cardiology
___ Lynch: Dermatology
___ MacFarlane: Urology
___ O'Donnell: Oncology
___ Pousada: Emergency Medicine
___ Rayburn: Obstetrics/Gynecology
___ Rudy: Family Medicine
___ Tisher: Nephrology
___ Tomb: Psychiatry
___ Vinetz: Infectious Disease
___ Waterbury: Hematology
___ Weiner: Neurology
___ Weiner: Pediatric Neurology
___ Wood: Radiology

Recall Series:
___ Bergin: Medicine Recall
___ Blackbourne: Surgical Recall
___ Blackbourne: Advanced Surgical Recall
___ Bourgeois: OB/GYN Recall
___ Fadem: Psychiatry Recall
___ Franko: Outpatient Medicine Recall
___ McGahren: Pediatrics Recall
___ Miller: Neurology Recall
___ Tribble: ICU Recall

Saint-Frances Series
Saint-Frances Guide to Inpatient Medicine
Saint-Frances Guide to Outpatient Medicine

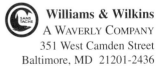
INTERNET:
E-mail: custserv@wwilkins.com
Home page: www.wwilkins.com
webROUNDS®: www.wwilkins.com/rounds

Printed in the US 997
CLERKADS ➡ 93345